# THE 10-DAY SKIN BRUSHING DETOX

# The 10-day

# SKIN

# BRUSHING

# DETOX

*The easy, natural plan to look great,*
*feel amazing, & eliminate cellulite*

**Mia Campbell**

Copyright © 2014 Mia Campbell

Second Edition

Coo Farm Press

First published January 2014 by Green Pony Press, Inc.

This edition published June 2014 by Coo Farm Press

Cambria and Times New Roman fonts used with permission from Microsoft.

**ISBN-10:** 0992960908 (Coo Farm Press)
**ISBN-13:** 978-0992960902

For Rosemary Jeffrey.

In loving memory of a life well lived.

# CONTENTS

⌘

# PREFACE

### ⚜

## *Somewhere in TV land*

THEY KNEW WHAT they wanted to do first after their huge lottery win. They booked into the ultimate luxury - the Golden Chamber spa.

Although they had dressed for the weather in comfortable shorts and t-shirts, it didn't help in the sweltering cab ride from the airport. Being multi-millionaires didn't help either. Even large amounts of cash can't fix broken air conditioning in a hurry. They arrived hot, frazzled, and sweating and were greeted by a snooty, suited, well-groomed woman who looked at them with horror and invited them to 'rinse off' before their assessment.

The assessment was a humiliating affair - they were forced to wear skin-tight leggings and leotards that hid nothing, and submit to the view of a superior woman assessing their 'faults'.

The spa's recommendations included cures for their thin hair, stubble, baggy skin, oddly-shaped breasts, sagging buttocks, and 'unpleasant fat'.

It seemed like a nightmare - a horror they had willingly paid for. And it got worse.

Massages included vigorous scrubbing with a large, stiff brush. They were given airtight, uncomfortable body wraps to purge their bodies of impurities, and body & bikini waxes that caused them to screech loudly enough to temporarily deafen themselves.

Then nutrition orders - NO dairy, NO sugar... no enjoyment.

Finally they were given an exercise schedule that left them feeling homicidal.

The result was to turn them off self-improvement and on to self-loathing - and want to order 2 pepperoni pizzas with extra toppings of 2 pepperoni pizzas.

Roseanne Conner and Jackie Harris had had enough. Health and vitality wasn't for them.

# How This Plan Can Revolutionize Your Health

CBEO

DESPITE BEING A fan of dry skin brushing, I laughed at the spa episode of the *Rosanne* TV show with everyone else in 1996. The episode was called 'Pampered to a Pulp' and portrayed skin brushing as an activity more suited to a torture chamber than a health spa.

I had qualified as an aromatherapist and massage therapist the year before, gaining diplomas from the International Institute of Health & Holistic Therapies and doing further study in nutrition (the nutrition courses were just out of interest, not to professional level).

None of my courses had covered skin brushing but my training made me realize that it would have many of the benefits of massage, plus some more, be quick and easy to do, and - unlike massage - would be easy to do yourself, without someone else doing the work.

I did experience the excellent results that skin brushing brings, but also suffered unfortunate side-effects. I couldn't find out any information about them, either online or in books or scientific papers. So I gave up daily brushing and just brushed occasionally.

When clients asked about skin brushing, I always advised them to be very careful. Brushing a healthy body is fine but when people with pre-existing illnesses take up brushing, they often become overwhelmed with negative side-effects.

A few years ago, I researched Manual Lymphatic Drainage (MLD). A close friend was battling cancer and MLD can help some of the painful swelling that can happen after lymph gland removal. I wanted to find out more about it before helping her find a therapist.

Now, if you read anything about skin brushing, the instructions will almost always say to start at the feet and work up, always brushing towards the heart. Some advise quite vigorous brushing. But MLD therapists don't start at the feet and they always use very gentle movements. Discovering that made a light bulb go off over my head! I had been doing skin brushing wrong for years.

Over a couple of months, I devised my own method, based on MLD principles and the effects I noticed. Then I started getting the people I massaged to try my method. They loved it and found that the effects spurred them on to continue brushing and to implement lifestyle changes.

There is no need for anyone to suffer with skin brushing and I'll show you how to take up the habit without succumbing to overwhelming side-effects that make you want to give up. You will find that skin brushing can kick-start a healthier lifestyle, because it gives you a glow, energy, and a new vibrancy that carries through into the rest of your life.

If you choose to **add** healthy foods, drinks, and habits to your life, instead of focusing on removing things, you will have an attitude of enjoyment and lack of stress. That feeling makes you feel WELL. Giving up stuff doesn't make you feel good; it puts your body into an alert mode, warning it that there's possible stress coming. The body starts putting stores of food into fat cells for later use, in case of famine; it cuts down on non-essential processes (such as copious energy, glossy hair, strong nails) and focuses on basic survival.

Natural energy – energy that comes from eating food that gives you nutrients, not food that uses them up – is amazing. It is nothing like the fake energy you get from chocolate or coffee. For a start, it lasts longer and doesn't leave you feeling even worse when the effects wear off because they don't wear off. There's also a kind of serenity that comes with natural energy that is hard to describe.

This skin brushing detox plan works as a type of diet because:

> Your new glow will make you feel less like cramming a whole chocolate cake into your mouth or reaching for your third glass of wine.

> You won't want to lose the healthy buzz so your body won't crave the old junk foods that used to give you a temporary lift but then a depressing fall-off.

> If you follow my recommendations about diet you will possibly be eating more than usual and that will make you feel less deprived, less stressed, and more at peace. You are far less likely to crave calorie dense, stodgy foods that feel like a lead lump in your stomach and sap your energy.

> You will be more relaxed and less stressed because you're doing something beneficial for your body.

> Dieting *isn't* the way to lose weight. Detoxing isn't either. The only way to lose weight is to get healthy. A healthy

body has no need of emergency stores of food, conveniently packaged in fat cells.

This book is about abundance and enjoyment. It's about taking up a new, enjoyable habit that makes you feel wonderful and then easing in some new health choices to support and nourish your mind and body.

It's about turning the word 'detox' on its head, realizing that we don't need to deprive ourselves in order to help our bodies go about their natural detoxification routines.

10 days are enough to give your body's natural detoxification systems a helping hand and to start you on the skin brushing habit. I was going to use the word 'addiction' instead of habit there, because that's what it's like. You feel so great that you won't want to miss a day!

After the 10 days, you could introduce another new habit or perhaps give up an old unhelpful habit, again for another 10 days. The 10 days thing is important because it takes that time for your body to adapt, to start to make it a habit, and to avoid clashing cleansing reactions. If you gave up caffeine, you'd probably get headaches. But if you gave up caffeine at the same time as taking up weight training, you couldn't be sure if it was the lack of caffeine or perhaps a pulled muscle in your neck causing the headaches.

You may not need a vast improvement in your health, you may just want a bit of a boost or smoother skin. Great. Long may it continue. It still applies that it is less stressful for your body if you take up new things one at a time though. If you have done skin brushing before you can just use this book to learn my new method and hopefully pick up some other tips as well.

The main thing I hope you will get out of this book is this:

## GO EASY

I'm pretty sure you won't believe me though, as skin brushing seems so simple and inoffensive. That's why the *Introduction* of this book goes into more detail about what happens when we deprive our bodies and *Chapter 1: My Story* details the side-effects that I experienced when I took up skin brushing. If you don't like personal stories then please feel free to skip it and go to *Chapter 2: A New Technique.*

Let's get started with a closer look at detoxing...

# PART ONE

---

# THE BASICS

# INTRODUCTION

❧

---

DEFINITION: **detox**

***A period when you stop taking unhealthy or
harmful foods, drinks, or drugs into
your body for a period of time, in order
to improve your health.***

Cambridge Dictionaries

---

I HAVE CALLED this book a detox plan but this is not like a traditional diet or detox. It isn't the type of detox where you give up lots of your usual food stuffs, suffer a whopping great headache, and spend most of your time groaning in the bathroom.

A detoxification is generally considered to be a removal of toxic substances - often alcohol or drugs. The modern use of the word 'detox' (the shortened term became popular in the 1970s) has been linked with alternative/complementary medicine.

Traditional doctors don't believe in the modern interpretation of the word 'detox' (not to be confused with clinical alcohol/drug detoxification). They don't think there is any need for what health writers call a detox, insisting that the body has its own detoxification organs and processes that don't require additional help.

I don't believe in detoxes either (detoxes where you give up lots of things and suffer from the effects of withdrawal from them, anyway). I don't believe in them because I have tried them and I've seen lots of other people try them and I've found that they don't work, especially long-term. Research has taught me why they don't work.

My plan is simple. It's just 10 days of supporting your body's natural detoxification systems via skin brushing, deep breathing, and rehydrating. Not giving things up, not suffering, and not putting unrealistic expectations on yourself.

It is a plan of abundance, not deprivation, because deprivation doesn't work. Deprivation of food - as proved in the Minnesota Starvation Experiment during World War II - causes horrendous problems, including:

➢ Decreased heart volume.
➢ Apathy & depression.
➢ Sensitivity to noise.
➢ Loss of ambition & narrowing of interests.
➢ Increased neuroticism & hysteria.
➢ Increased interest & preoccupation with food.
➢ Heightened craving for food.
➢ Reduction of humor & tolerance.
➢ Increased self-centeredness.
➢ Inability to control emotions.

Similar to the things a lot of people go through when dieting today.

If you've heard of it at all, you may think that the Minnesota Starvation Experiment involved complete starvation, or fasting. It didn't. The participants merely ate a reduced calorie diet - which contained MORE calories than many modern crash diets – but they weren't sitting around, they were doing some work.

They ate just under half their usual calorie intake for 6 months. This amount was determined by the investigators after observing them eating normally for the previous 3 months.

The Minnesota experiment used volunteers - who were conscientious objectors - to find out what effects famine had on the human body. They needed to know, to determine how to provide relief assistance to famine victims of the war. After the experiment was over it took 33 weeks for the participants to return to normal eating, sleeping, and social behavior and their previous humor 'slowly returned'.

For the sake of clarity, allow me to repeat that. They ate HALF of their usual calories. The volunteers were all healthy men, and their controlled diet caloric intake before the 'starvation' was an average of 3,200 daily (depending on their weight). During the 'starvation' the men ate an average of 1,560 calories each day. **1,560**. That is more than is recommended by many modern diets, a lot more than recommended by some diets (LighterLife recommends just 500-600 calories a day in the initial phase).

The volunteers became obsessed with food during the starvation phase. Their behavior became irrational and uncontrolled. One man actually chopped off three of his fingers with an axe. He later said: "I admit to being crazy mixed up. As of 50 years later, I am not ready to say I did it on purpose. I am not ready to say I didn't."

This sounds like the deliberate self-harm that anorexics go through. Or the passive-aggressive self-harm through drinking, smoking, and drug taking of unhappy models and others who have to remain unnaturally slim.

Do we really want to do this to ourselves? Is a crash diet to lose some weight worth the risk of putting our heart in trouble, alienating friends & family, putting our job security in jeopardy, losing our sense of humor, and more?

The Minnesota experiment produced another effect. Many of the men ended up binging heavily once the experiment was over. Like many of us do when we 'fall off the wagon' when dieting. We swing from starving ourselves to binging and back again. Often, we do this throughout our lives. Perhaps not in as extreme a manner as undergone by the volunteers in the experiment, but if we don't provide our bodies with the calories and nutrients that they need, we will experience the same negative effects, just in a lesser way that takes longer to show the worst of its effects.

The Minnesota experiment demonstrated that people who have endured a period of starvation need up to 5,000 calories a day to recover from it. Not vitamin or protein mixtures, just real food and lots of it. Those of us who have experimented with various diets and detoxes over the years have been responsible for putting ourselves through stress not unlike that suffered by people in war zones. Your body thinks there's a war going on. And you wonder why you're finding it hard to resist food cravings? Your body could be starving for various nutrients and doing whatever it can to get you to eat to get them.

Let's look at what happens when we don't eat enough. Our body will assume something dreadful is happening - such as war or famine (or our agreeing to take part in a starvation experiment!). The body starts to focus on staying alive and won't 'waste' valuable resources (calories/nutrients) on things that aren't essential to life. So no more glossy hair, strong nails, soft skin, bright eyes. And lots of anxiety, depression, loss of concentration, etc.

Many of us live in that state of pseudo famine almost all our lives. Instead of enjoying vibrant health, we have to buy expensive moisturizers to make our faces look less washed out, nail treatments to try to stop our nails flaking and breaking, various drugs and addictions to give us energy (caffeine, sugar) or calm us down enough to be able to sleep (drugs, herbal tranquillizers, other sleep aids - legal and otherwise).

I put it to you that it's time to give your body, your mind, and your spirit a break. It's time to let your body know that you care for it and are going to give it what it needs. Real food. Healthy habits. Care and support.

It's time to let your mind know that you no longer expect it to function on less than adequate nutrition (the brain uses about 300 calories a day - unless it is thinking very hard, when it burns through more); on negative, self-hating thoughts; on stressful, anxious matters.

It's time to let your spirit know that you recognize its existence. You don't have to be religious to acknowledge that you have a spirit.

One last thing before we leave the topic of the Minnesota Starvation Experiment. The main investigator, nutritionist Ancel Keys (who went on to discover the link between cholesterol and heart disease), followed a Mediterranean-type diet - lots of vegetables, olive oil, red wine, fish. That is a diet of abundance and enjoyment. He lived an active life with lots of good food, swimming, and walking. He died at the age of 100 in 2004. He remained a scientist right to the end. Asked at his 100th birthday party if his Mediterranean diet was the reason for his longevity, he said: "Very likely, but no proof."

I found out about Ancel Keys and the Minnesota Starvation Experiment when, in desperation, I took my daughter - who was suffering terribly with the effects of anorexia - to see the well-known UK nutritionist Zoe Harcombe. She sat my daughter in a warm, cozy spot in her kitchen - knowing that anorexics are permanently freezing due to lack of caloric intake. Zoe didn't demand that my daughter explain herself as to why she wasn't eating, knowing that she would be unable to formulate the sentences due to lack of brain food. She just gently told us her own life story, about her battles with anorexia and bulimia and how she overcame them.

She explained about the Minnesota Starvation Experiment and the fact that people need 1,500 calories a day just for basic bodily functions. You need that amount even if you're lying in bed all day, when you add in normal daily activities, work, exercise, study, etc., you need more (much more, in many cases).

My daughter and I realized that, like many other people (women in particular), we had both been putting ourselves through our own mini versions of the Minnesota Starvation Experiment. I had been doing it via various detoxes and diets for over 40 years. My daughter had been doing it via anorexia. Anorexia for her, and for many sufferers, was a crutch to support her through a difficult time. It was her way of coping with something else.

Trying to remove anorexia is like trying to remove the crutch from a person with one leg, who relies on it for walking. Not a good idea. But when the crutch itself is life-threatening, it's time to find a better crutch, or find a way to do without a crutch completely.

Working with Zoe taught us that we needed to become healthy in order to get better. That might sound like an odd way of putting it but it was a phrase similar to one I heard later on from another of my heroes, Dr Eric Berg, who is a US chiropractor and weight loss expert. He says you shouldn't diet to lose weight, you should get healthy to lose weight. If you aren't healthy enough, your body won't be willing to let go of its emergency food rations that it has so carefully stored in your fat cells.

The story of my life-long battle for health is in Chapter One. If you don't like long stories, you can skip it. I'll put it in a nutshell here:

> Years of quite serious ill health after being in a car wreck, followed by multiple surgeries.
> Yo-yo attempts at dieting, detoxing, and trying to get fit and healthy.
> Failure and defeat only to try again and fail again - with my weight getting heavier and my health getting worse all the time.

For many years, I was either dieting or binging. When I dieted I was in a state of starvation, of deprivation. When I was off a diet I was in a state of abundance, eating anything I liked, enjoying life. Well, for a while, as eating everything you want makes you feel ill eventually if what you want is unhealthy food!

It's a pretty normal story really. Many people do it every New Year's Eve. We make resolutions to fix the things that have been bothering us. We often do it in such an 'all-or-nothing' way, though, that it is impossible to keep up. Then we give up, defeated, sometime in early January, convincing ourselves that we aren't capable of sticking to anything.

When I discovered a naturopathic technique that had terrific effects, I went at it the way I had done all the diet/health things I tried before - with devastating side-effects. So I gave it up.

Dry skin brushing (I'll call it skin brushing from now on but I always mean brushing that is done with a dry brush on dry skin) is a very simple yet very powerful technique that can be used on its own to improve health, increase lymphatic and blood circulation, tackle cellulite, increase energy, and much more. What it does is give you a glow, a healthy vibrancy that makes you want to eat better and even think better. It helps take you out of the starvation phase of your own personal Minnesota Starvation Experiment and into the recovery phase. The phase of returning to enjoying life, of returning to a healthy weight, of not being obsessed with food or diets or health.

During the recovery phase, the experiment volunteers naturally ate more calories because their bodies knew that the nutrients were needed for rebuilding themselves. After around 15 weeks of eating many more calories than they would have if they hadn't been through the starvation phase, their social behavior started to return to normal. By week 20 they nearly all felt normal around food. By week 33 they had returned to eating normal amounts and no longer binged. Touchingly, the investigators noticed that humor returned.

What does all that have to do with you? Well I imagine that you've been beating up on yourself in one way or another. Perhaps through diets and detoxes, or through negative thinking, exercise (or lack of it), alcohol, drugs, overwork. Humans are really creative, we can think of lots of ways to self-destruct!

This little book can help you to stop beating yourself up. It can do that by introducing you to a really quick, easy, effective health technique called skin brushing. Done improperly, though, skin brushing can cause headaches, joint pain, brain fog, nausea, and skin irritation. Those sorts of feelings make you reach for stimulants to make you feel better - caffeine, alcohol, sugar, fats. Once you do, you crave more and it's the old downward spiral to ill-health again.

The definition of detox is a period of giving up harmful things – usually thought to be just food and drinks. Maybe it could also include giving up harmful thoughts too, especially those directed at ourselves.

So I hope you will use the techniques in this book and the advice I heap on in shovelfuls not to take it too quickly or go at it like a bull in a china shop that's located on the way to a field of fertile cows.

Go easy. Go easy on the technique and on yourself. Whatever state you're in, you are actually a work of art, a miracle of biology. For you to have made it through conception, pregnancy, and birth was a fantastic, amazing achievement. Everything else is just detail.

# Chapter 1
## My Story

ಆಹಿ

A S I DROVE to work on a country road I was happily singing along to a song on the radio. Seconds later, a speeding car driven by a hobby rally driver overtook several other cars on a blind bend and smashed into me doing over 60mph.

Several things went very right, despite so much going wrong. The police, ambulance, and fire engine got there quickly. Among the people who stopped to help was a high court judge (who made a terrific witness in the court case that followed). The impact happened outside an animal shelter. These places are run, naturally, by very caring people and the owner was a particular star. She rushed out to help, comforting me and trying to decipher what I was mumbling through a face full of smashed bones. She could only make out a few words, my husband's name and the large, national company he worked for.

When the police and ambulance people took over, she dashed to a telephone and spoke to what must have been dozens of people before she located someone in the company who had heard of my husband. As a result, my husband and mother (he rang her as soon as he heard) were at the hospital before I even got there (it took them a while to cut me out of my wrecked car). Funny how things can go right while they're also going wrong.

Before the accident I was youthfully healthy and fit. I loved badminton, yoga, swimming, dog training, and horseback riding. I was a healthy and muscular size 2-4 when I got married in 1986 and stayed that size even after starting to eat man-sized meals with my new husband, as I was happy and active.

After the accident - where my ankles were crushed, amongst numerous other injuries - I was unable to do all the active things I had done before. Once the shock and pain started to ease, I began to feel frustrated at the lack of movement. My legs were in large, heavy plaster casts and one arm was strapped up. I had internal injuries and was scared to move as everything hurt so much.

My jaws were wired together and all I could eat was a 'high nutrition' liquid that the hospital prescribed. Despite being unable to eat properly, I didn't lose a pound during the months my jaws were wired. The drink was a combination of sugar and fat. My inability to move meant that my metabolism crashed too.

My frustration spilled over into moaning so my husband and dad bought me an exercise bike that they lifted me onto twice a day. I was delighted that this meant that I wouldn't lose muscle mass from all the lying around. When the plaster casts were removed my calves were as toned as before. So the cycling did some good, even if it didn't help me lose any weight!

Unfortunately, the removal of the casts meant the end of my cycling fun. My ankles were floppy and unstable and pedaling hurt, a lot. I started to put weight on as walking and other exercise was prohibitively painful too.

Worse, I was unable to get pregnant. We tried for several years but were finally told we were unlikely to have children due to the problems caused to my inner plumbing by the accident.

To learn about how to get healthy, I bought some health books (any excuse to buy books!). I cleaned up my diet, added home-made [vegetable] juices, smoothies, and yogurt, and removed processed, high-fat, and high-sugar foods. My husband was resistant to dietary change so I was more sneaky with his food (don't judge me - we needed healthy sperm!), adding green leaves to the fruit-based smoothies that he loved, making bread (lower salt than bought bread and boosted with iron-rich molasses and oil-loaded ground seeds) and biscuits (lower sugar and fat and no hydrogenated fats).

My parents had conceived me after giving up trying and deciding to take a great vacation - blowing the money they had been saving up for a baby. They went abroad and relaxed in the sun, forgetting all the stress of the previous years and disappointment with not being able to conceive. Nine months later, I arrived. Relaxation and freedom from worry seems to really matter when you're trying to get pregnant.

So my husband and I booked some vacations. We were thinking of giving up trying to have a family of our own and emigrating to the US to live with my husband's brother, who had married an American girl and had a son and baby daughter. I figured if I couldn't have my own babies I would concentrate on being an aunt. So we booked a flight to Atlanta, Georgia for October 1991.

Before that, we had a week's vacation in August at a cottage within the grounds of a manor house in the beautiful Cotswolds in England. The owners were friendly and welcoming. They told us they were in the middle of a Christian meeting in their home and invited us to join in. It was a living room full of local people with shared Christian beliefs but who weren't keen on traditional churches. It was a charmingly relaxed hour or so with worship led by a superbly-talented pair of blind musicians.

None of the people knew we were trying to conceive. I mean, we weren't making out in the corner or anything and I wasn't chugging vitamin pills and refusing the communion wine.

Everyone was offered prayer. I tried to remain British about it, polite and non-emotional, but the stress of the previous years - the accident, the operations to rebuild various bits of me, the stress of not being able to get pregnant, money worries, and more - came out in a deluge of tears. When I was dehydrated enough to stop, I felt better. So did my husband, who had been through it all too and couldn't watch me cry without joining in.

We had a blissful vacation. Our dog Rocky was much admired by the locals, which made his week. We enjoyed spending time together away from our busy work schedules. We explored the Cotswold villages and vegged out after stuffing ourselves with superb locally-grown produce.

Nine months later, Josh was born.

Was it the improvement in my diet? Was it the relaxation? Was it God, the power of prayer? I am convinced that it was all three combined. I have a body, a soul, and a spirit - I had only been taking care of my body up until then. I had been focusing my diet on what I **shouldn't** be eating. I had been focusing on problems, on feeling a victim, feeling deprived, stressing myself out. Afterwards I focused on possibilities, relaxation, hope.

There would have been no good in eating a superb diet if my insides had been completely scrunched up with worry and stress - I wouldn't have absorbed all the nutrients.

There would have been no good if I was so chilled out and relaxed that I didn't take care with my diet or health - my body wouldn't have had the nutrients it needed to cope with or start the process of pregnancy.

There would have been no good in eating a good diet and being relaxed if I had remained convinced that the doctors were right and I would never conceive. If I didn't believe that somehow my ravaged body could be renewed to make it capable of enduring a pregnancy I honestly don't think I would ever have got pregnant.

There's a lot of talk about holistics, things working together.

I get it.

ଔଞ୍ଚ

Josh was a couple of months old – fat, gorgeous and a happy baby (now a happy, 6' 3" just-married man) - when I decided to consult a herbalist. I was still breastfeeding so didn't want to take pharmaceutical drugs but I was suffering from depression (probably post-natal but could have been caused by the knock on the head during the accident) and needed help.

I felt overweight, now up to a size 8 from a 2-4. I had no energy and no inclination to do anything about generating energy. My ankles were still painful so swimming was one of the few exercises I could do without having to resort to industrial-strength painkillers. But taking a baby swimming was such a huge effort that I felt I would have benefited from training in project management. The most I could manage was packing the nappy bag, slinging it on the stroller, and taking a short walk to local shops – being lapped by other mothers with strollers who seemed to be in some sort of race that no-one had told me about.

I had read a book by Kitty Campion, a herbalist who has written extensively on women's health issues. A bit of research revealed that she lived (then) in Stoke-on-Trent, a 2-hour drive from my home. I made an appointment.

Kitty is a calm, self-assured woman with a herbal database in her brain and a deep desire to help others. She diagnosed me by using (among other things) iridology, a way of assessing the health of the body through the irises of the eye. I wasn't too sure about iridology. It isn't recognized by medical science and is seen as something 'quack' doctors do. But quack doctors don't tend to drive top-of-the-range Mercedes, spend a lot of their working week on golf courses, or lose large numbers of their patients due to pharmaceutical drugs. Plus, iridology isn't invasive or too weird so I was prepared to give it a go.

I now prefer [carefully-researched and selected] 'quack' doctors. Medical science managed to keep me alive after my accident (although there were times when the pain or depression got too much that I inwardly criticized them for doing so) but they hadn't restored me to health. They stitched me back together and thought that was enough. It wasn't.

Kitty asked me not to tell her anything about my problems. She sat me at a setup like you would see in an optometrist's office. I rested my chin on a little shelf and stared into the contraption; she sat the other side and looked at my irises.

What she saw in my eyes was that my ankles had been fractured, my right clavicle broken, my bowel displaced, my jaws fractured, and other results of the accident. I was amazed. She went on to say that she was worried about my lymphatic system, which appeared to be very sluggish, and my mental health.

That was when she looked up at me over the top of the video-camera-scope-thing. She held my gaze and asked me where the unendurable stress in my life was coming from. She said if I didn't get on top of the stress (she suggested learning to be assertive, learn how to say no, and start taking positive action in my thoughts and in my life), I was doomed to a - probably short - life of ill-health. She prescribed a number of things but stressed that they would only tackle some of my symptoms - and even many of those had been caused by stress and mental issues. It left me with a lot to think about.

The next day I started the skin brushing that Kitty recommended. I plunged right into it and did it vigorously, twice daily. Kitty also suggested several diet and lifestyle changes and I began those by cutting out tea – on the same day.

I stuck to it really well... for about a day and a half. I got the worst headache known to man and nothing would shift it. Kitty had warned me it was possible - a side-effect of giving up caffeine - but as I hadn't been a coffee drinker I didn't think I would be affected. Kitty suggested drinking more water and taking some gentle exercise. I felt too sick to try either.

People under-estimate the awfulness of caffeine withdrawal. Yet caffeine is a huge problem in our society - a powerful drug that is socially acceptable. I was lucky I was **only** a tea drinker - it's even worse for coffee drinkers when they try to give up.

My follow-up appointment revealed that the crushing headache wasn't just from caffeine withdrawal, but a side-effect of skin brushing. When you brush your skin you stimulate the lymph that flows beneath it. Mobilizing the lymphatic system is a good thing but lymph is responsible for getting rid of a lot of the junk in your body – e.g. dead cells and toxins - and you don't want a load of those suddenly released and flooding your system. It didn't seem possible that something so simple could have such a powerful effect. But it did.

The combination of side-effects continued. They seemed to affect my immune system and I succumbed to a nasty cold. Healthy eating went out of the window as I craved ice-cream for my sore throat. I gave up skin brushing while I languished in bed - and didn't get back into it as I wasn't able to afford to go back to Kitty (who would have motivated me to keep going).

Not long after, we went on vacation to Devon. It's a surfer's paradise and those of us who are incapable of keeping their balance even on dry land just enjoy watching them. It was another vacation that was memorable for its wonderfulness. The British weather, for once, was good and we visited a lot of fun places with Josh, who was now a just-toddling one-year-old. We spent much of the week laughing at his reactions to the various animals he was seeing for the first time. A great week.

So it was a surprise but not a total shock to find out that I was pregnant a few weeks later. The pregnancy went well - I always feel at my best when flooded with pregnancy hormones - and I was looking forward to the birth. Seriously. I love giving birth. OK, it's painful but the unique act of taking part in creation, of bringing forth an actual human being, someone who had previously existed only in your mind, is a supreme privilege and worth the pain. Although that could be the gas & air talking!

This birth was different. My husband had a nervous breakdown just before I was due. A total breakdown. A sobbing on the floor, unable to get up, staring vacantly into space type of breakdown.

He was at the birth - the difficult birth as our daughter weighed 11lb 8.5oz and wasn't in any hurry to leave the womb. I was grateful for his presence as I knew it required huge effort on his part. But he wasn't really there, only physically. He left the hospital after holding his baby briefly and I was left bereft. To say he never really recovered would be an exaggeration but only slightly. He never returned to the cheerful person he had been.

Life after that was plagued with illness and stress. Coping with pain myself, money problems, work problems (my husband had an accident at work and was coping with severe back pain but wasn't covered by insurance and wasn't allowed any more sick leave), my husband's OCD (which affected all of us and limited our activities), and the struggles of bringing up young children.

C3&0

What does all that whining have to do with a book about skin brushing? Everything.

Fast forward 10 years. All this time I was eating a superb, healthy diet. I took high quality supplements, avoided tea & coffee, never touched soda. Yet I was ill. I was unable to cope with basic household tasks and rarely able to manage the short walk to the shops. Eventually I was diagnosed with Chronic Fatigue Syndrome.

I saw a number of health professionals - traditional and complementary - including a doctor who had CFS. He told me I had an overgrowth of Candida in my body. He recommended daily swims in the ocean (not practical - he lived on the coast, I didn't) and a very restricted diet. So I followed an anti-Candida diet. I had tried one before, just after Josh was born, but had had to give it up due to the impracticalities, side-effects, and the general busyness of new motherhood.

The 'die-off' symptoms this time were as bad as when I had first started skin brushing. Flooding my body with dying Candida wasn't the smartest thing to do. I started doing a little careful skin brushing (I knew from experience to take it slowly) and took up gentle rebounding to help move the rubbish out of my body. That helped. I was eating well, taking supplements and exercising as much as I was able to. Yet I was still ill.

I had qualified as a Massage Therapist & Aromatherapist the year after my daughter was born, and I took a course on nutrition as well. My training had included anatomy and physiology so I understood the human body and thought that knowledge would help me recover.

I started to look back through old diaries and took notes. The only times in my life post-accident, that I had felt well had been: a) on vacation and b) when pregnant and/or breastfeeding.

Staying pregnant and/or being permanently on vacation weren't feasible options. Especially considering what happened next.

My husband and I split up. I was very involved with setting up a training franchise that we were just starting as a family business and he felt abandoned. He was at university at the time and he met someone else there. We had signed leases and contracts so I had no option but to try to make the business work, despite feeling like I was dying inside emotionally. I missed him. I still loved him and hoped he would come back. But he never did and I agreed to his request for a divorce.

Josh had left college by this time and joined me in the business. He was superb. He was great with the students, good at solving computer problems, and brilliant at covering for me when I was ill. Which I was, more and more. We struggled on for two years before calling it a day. It was a training franchise that had seemed ideal for my skills but what they actually needed were franchisees with very strong selling skills (although they didn't tell me that, these people never do!). Despite me not having any selling skills, they had happily sold me the (expensive) franchise.

I was never going to be happy or good at selling people courses they either couldn't afford or didn't really need. It went against my integrity to recommend a course costing thousands of dollars when a shorter one costing hundreds would get the person the job they wanted. Perhaps I could have done it if I had known it would help them get a job but in the recession jobs were very scarce.

We tried to close 6 months before we finally managed it. The franchisor kept asking us to hang on and assuring us they would find a buyer for the business. We were terrified of closing the door and walking away because they made it clear that they had the right to sue us for loss of earnings for the remainder of the franchise agreement.

We also didn't want to let our students down. We provided a safe haven for them that was very unlike the hustle and bustle of a traditional college and they thrived. But we were getting an additional $2,000 deeper in debt every month and we had to close, despite knowing that it would plunge us even more into debt due to being no longer able to contribute to leases and loans. My health was giving out alarmingly and I agreed to close the business after my children sat me down and told me they didn't want to lose another parent.

The following years were a nightmare of debt, legal letters, credit records, and court appearances. Fear of the mail arriving became part of our lives and we had a family cheer of "No bad post" on good days and white-faced panic on bad days. My daughter, who had been battling anorexia for a number of years, became desperately, worryingly ill and had to leave college.

During this bleak time, though, a miracle happened. I met Andrew. We had so much it common it was ridiculous. Andrew is a writer & musician, he'd also had an accident (motorbike), also has facial scars (his covered with a gorgeous, glossy beard), loves herbal teas, loves dogs and hens, and much more.

He looked past my scars, insecurities, and hurts. He saw the real me, the one struggling to get out.

Andrew was a turning point in my life in more ways than I probably even now realize. He was confident and liked himself. It was possible to like yourself without being a diva?! Huh, who knew?

He was calm and relaxing to be around yet very capable - he fitted a tow bar to Josh's car in a couple of hours and restored lighting and electricity to our garage. All without drama and stress.

I found myself becoming less stressed. Well, after realizing what a screeching harpy I could be at times as it was such a contrast to his perpetual air of calm.

His father had been a Methodist minister, so he had grown up with a faith that he now lived. Not in a Bible-thumping, evangelical kind of way, but in a quiet, "God's in control, it'll all work out for the best" kind of way.

I had rid myself of most of the problems of CFS using a method that is mainly mind-based, the Lightning Process, the year before we met. (That isn't to say that CFS is all in the mind. But I knew for certain that how I thought about things, how stressed I allowed myself to get, and how rigid I got about my diet negatively affected how I felt. So I knew that using a method of getting thought processes in line and using thoughts in a positive way rather than letting them come and go at will was going to help and stop the adrenaline highs and lows that made the CFS pain worse.) I now understood why I had more energy since meeting Andrew - it was because I was happy and my thoughts weren't going down their old negative tracks.

But I was still in a lot of pain and very restricted. Being unable to do things you love - I miss horseback riding SO much - tends to leave you feeling inadequate and moody.

Andrew is also in pain and also restricted in what he can do physically. But I've rarely seen him in a bad mood. Hmm.

He's in superb physical health, despite taking very strong painkillers daily, having limited liver function, and suffering from fibromyalgia. Hmm.

I started to wonder about the whole health thing again. My diet had gone downhill after my divorce (I stress eat - and chocolate can lift a mood like nothing else! - plus I had got hooked on Diet Pepsi while suffering from CFS) and I was overweight but the more time I spent around Andrew, the better I felt for his calming influence. He ate a healthy diet most of the time but didn't fret if he chose a big piece of chocolate cake when having a meal out. He drank mostly herbal teas but started each day with a STRONG cup of coffee and didn't worry about getting hooked on caffeine. He exercised but would happily laze away a day at the beach without fearing he was becoming a couch potato (beach potato?!).

I had a revelation. A complete epiphany. Every time I had tried to improve my health, I had done it with an all-or-nothing approach, all at the same time. I would do a total detox, giving up sugar and fat completely; suddenly starting to exercise every day; doing skin brushing twice a day; adopting an extreme diet; avoiding caffeine completely.

The result was a rush of toxins in my bloodstream, headaches, nausea, joint pain, and other horrible side-effects. I would get overwhelmed, feel inadequate, give up EVERYTHING, and collapse into bed.

I realized I didn't have to give up the amazing benefits that skin brushing gives - I just needed to do it like Andrew would do if he took it up. He would start gently, get into the swing of it, and enjoy it without fretting if he missed the odd day. He wouldn't take up another habit at the same time, he'd get used to one on its own.

I understood that my history of taking up healthy habits all at once had always been doomed to disaster, because I did them so stressily. I did them in the hope that they would solve all the other problems in my life, wipe away all the stress. But I was just adding yet another stressor! I did them with a 'This has to work or I'm done for' attitude. No matter how healthy those habits were, they wouldn't have done me any good because my insides were in a perpetual knot due to stress. So I wasn't digesting the good food I ate, wasn't absorbing enough nutrients, wasn't getting the benefit out of lifestyle changes because my negative thoughts were poisoning my mind and body.

I made a plan for myself. A re-introduction to healthy habits that started with skin brushing, because I knew from past experience that that had a very quick effect and would encourage me to keep going and take up other good health habits.

I did it. It was easy. I didn't end up with vile headaches and other side-effects. I was encouraged by my success and gradually took up other healthy habits.

I started to lose weight without feeling deprived, or it leaving me with sagging skin. I toned up my skin and muscles just by skin brushing initially. I no longer suffer from mood swings. I lost my taste for overly-sweet foods and my craving for stodge.

It was so easy. Well, it was after I decided to stop stressing about life, the universe, and everything.

After I decided to like and accept myself.

After I decided to stop pummeling my body with harsh diets and regimes and instead take up new health habits gently.

It all started with skin brushing. But not skin brushing as you may have come across it before...

# CHAPTER 2
# A NEW TECHNIQUE

CB⅏

D R EMIL VODDER was born in 1896 in Copenhagen. He was something of a Renaissance man with an incredible capacity for learning - studying 10 languages, biology, mineralology, botany, medicine, cytology, and microscopy. He was also an accomplished singer and cellist.

He was studying to be a doctor when he became very ill with malaria and was never able to finish his medical degree, although he retained a passionate interest in physical medicine. He earned the right to the title of 'doctor' when he was awarded a PhD following the publication of his thesis on Historical Art.

He had married a naturopath, Estrid, and became very interested in the body's lymphatic system, studying scientific papers and the little medical wisdom there was then on the subject. He became convinced that the lymphatic system is the most important system in the human (and animal) body.

Emil started to treat patients - presumably Estrid's - who were suffering from swollen lymph glands. These patients often had acne, migraines, or sinus problems, which Emil believed were caused by the swollen lymph glands - not the other way around (i.e. not the acne causing the swollen lymph glands). This was revolutionary thought.

He believed that unblocking the nodes would be like opening the floodgates of a dam - the lymph glands would be able to carry out their work of cleansing the tissues and the related problems would be helped. He started to try out techniques for encouraging the blocked and swollen lymph glands to drain. He wondered if it was possible to massage them clear.

It is hard for us in the 21st century to understand what a pioneer Emil was. In those days even doctors didn't dare to touch swollen glands. Not enough was known about them. Yet Emil was massaging them, using gentle circling, stretching movements to decongest the nodes and improve the related health conditions. His patients' illnesses - acne, colds, migraines, sinuses - cleared when their swollen lymph glands drained.

In 1933 he and Estrid moved to Paris and Emil was delighted to discover a collection of copper engravings by the anatomist Sappey, which further enhanced his understanding of the lymphatic system. He and Estrid developed the technique and it eventually became what we now know as Manual Lymphatic Drainage (MLD). It was used to treat the body as a whole, not just an afflicted part, although Emil would give extra attention to an afflicted area.

Emil was ahead of his time, complaining that, "I discovered my method too early. No-one understands me." Yet years later his technique is used by, among others, the German Health System and the National Health Service in the UK. German health insurance companies refund payments for MLD, in fact it is the most frequently prescribed manual technique that doctors use in Germany.

People who met and worked with Emil said he was a brilliant, funny, humble, and liberal man. He refused to make money from his life's work but finally accepted recognition from the German Massage and Physical Therapy Association, who acknowledged him as the creator of the method they called 'Dr Vodder's Manual Lymph Drainage'.

MLD didn't arrive in the US until 1972 and a Vodder School was founded in 1993. MLD is now a very respected 'skin technique'* that is recommended for, amongst other things, post-cancer surgery and/or when people are afflicted with lymphedema[1]. When cancer spreads (or metastases) it often does so via the lymphatic system[2] and, as a result, lymph glands can become cancerous. The affected nodes have to be removed but that can then result in a build-up of lymphatic fluid around the area because the usually hard-working node which processes the fluid is missing. Tissue can become very swollen and painful. MLD is a gentle technique that moves the fluid along and can also teach the lymph that there are other - healthy - vessels that it can go through.

MLD therapists know a lot about the lymphatic system - the system that we are primarily working with when we practice skin brushing. But there's a huge difference in how MLD therapists work and how most people say you should do skin brushing.

When I get into a subject I like to read up a lot about it. Frustratingly, when I got interested in skin brushing I wasn't able to find a book devoted to it and the Internet didn't exist in those days. I was limited to reading the odd passage in health books. Notable were Kitty Campion's herbal books, Leslie

---

1 If you have lymphedema there is some excellent advice on: www.lymphnet.org.
2 The other methods of cancer spreading are via the blood vessels or body cavities.

Kenton's books on raw food and other health topics, and Dr Ross Trattler's naturopathic book, 'Better Health Through Natural Healing'.

I wanted to learn more than the basics - the basics being that skin brushing is great for exfoliation, skin tone, blood circulation, and cellulite. Even the tutors on my massage & aromatherapy courses didn't know more than that.

My patience was rewarded when I came across MLD - and I was shocked. I realized that everybody was giving the wrong advice when it comes to skin brushing. Every skin brushing article, passage, or video I have seen has instructed people to start at the feet. I guess it makes sense in a way because the feet are the furthest body part from the heart so you would think that you want to encourage the circulation there to travel back up the legs. So far so good. But wrong because one of the huge benefits of skin brushing is its effect on the lymphatic system.

Think about a piping bag used to ice cakes. If that stuff gets good and packed in there and dries up and you can't wash it out would you try to squeeze it out by squeezing from the end of the bag? That wouldn't work it if was really blocked. It would take a tremendous amount of pressure to shift it and you would run the risk of the bag bursting. You would need to encourage it out a bit at a time by squeezing near the nozzle, right near the top, getting a bit out at a time, then working your way down the bag gradually. Getting some water in there would help, too.

It's the same with manual lymphatic drainage. Therapists generally start at the top, in the area where the processed lymph drains back into the venus system in the upper chest – not at the feet. They work their hands with a light stretching motion[3] near and towards that drain, then move them a little way back and work toward the drain again. It's the same on the arm. They start at the nearest collection of healthy lymph glands, stretching the skin gently towards them then moving a little way back and stretching towards the lymph glands again, a bit at a time.

Most people, when recommending skin brushing, will tell you to brush everything from below the heart upwards and everything from above the heart downwards. But this isn't what MLD therapists do.

MLD is a very gentle, specialist technique but we can copy the movements and gain some of the same effects with our skin brushing - and make it a far more effective treatment for the all-important lymphatic system than if we did it the way everybody else tells us to, from the feet up.

That's how I've created this plan, by learning from the movements of various MLD methods to make this the most effective skin brushing technique ever.

The simple thing to remember is this: Whichever part of the body you are working on, you are working towards the nearest group of [healthy] nodes that drain that area, and you are going to work nearest the nodes first, moving away but still towards them, gradually.

Let's look at the amazing benefits you will get out of it...

---

3 Vodder-trained MLD therapists don't call it massage, they call it a skin technique. Massage involves deeper work, MLD is very light and gentle.

# CHAPTER 3
# THE BENEFITS OF SKIN BRUSHING

CRSEO

**M**Y INTRODUCTION TO dry skin brushing was in Kitty Campion's book, 'Holistic Woman's Herbal'. It contained lots of benefits of dry skin brushing. So many that they almost aren't believable but it turns out that Kitty had been brief in her version of the benefits! It is one of the cheapest, most effective things you can do to improve your health and it takes just a couple of minutes a day.

Far from skin brushing being an over-hyped fad, the technique is a well-known naturopathic method of healing that gives both immediate and long-term results... if done properly.

If not, and if you go about it like I did initially - too much, too quickly - you could find the side-effects extremely uncomfortable, which could put you off doing it. That would be a pity, because this technique could improve your health tremendously.

So let's start by encouraging ourselves and looking at all the benefits that dry skin brushing can bring. Remember, these are real benefits, reported by thousands of people who have nothing to gain by reporting them; and I have experienced most of them myself.

It can help to refer back to this chapter if ever you feel like skipping your daily brushing!

## IMMEDIATE/VERY QUICK BENEFITS

- Improvement in skin's appearance and texture.
- Improved muscle tone.
- Improved lymphatic movement. You may not realize this is what is happening but you will notice your complexion clearing up if you suffer from acne, less sinus problems, less pain in the armpits, less dragging pain in the legs.
- More energy.

## LATER BENEFITS

- Reduction of cellulite. Many people do skin brushing just to get rid of cellulite, it is well known to be very effective.
- Improved immunity.
- Improved muscle tone.
- Less fatty deposits.
- Improved skin condition.
- Better varicose veins.
- Better digestion.
- Improved hormones.
- A feeling of wellbeing and an inner and outer glow of vibrant energy.

This may seem far-fetched, so don't believe me - try it for yourself! Read on, too, to understand a bit more about the different body systems and how they are improved by skin brushing.

# THE SKIN

Skin cells are constantly renewing and the old ones near the surface are supposed to slough off, revealing the newer skin underneath. In practice, they often don't all fall off without a bit of help. Our skin seems to get less able to renew itself without help as we get older, and during times of ill health and in winter (when we cover it up from head to toe to keep warm). Skin brushing gets rid of the dead skin cells almost overnight. Your skin not only looks better, it feels soft and smooth. Almost like a baby's beautiful skin.

This is the effect that we are all looking for when we buy AHA creams for our complexions. They stimulate cell renewal, remove dead skin cells and reveal a brighter, fresher complexion. For around $50 a pot!

You can get the same effect through GENTLE skin brushing of your face, neck and décolleté. I have found that skin brushing does definitely and quickly stimulate cell renewal. If you accompany your skin brushing with taking EFAs (essential fatty acids, which sound slightly more palatable than 'fats' or 'oils' don't you think?!), it will have an even more striking effect.

Skin brushing even encourages collagen production - another thing we generally pay a lot of money for little pots of creams to do.

## THE ELIMINATION CONNECTION

The skin is overlooked by many people as being just an outer covering for the more important bodily organs. In fact the skin IS an organ and it is one of the most important elimination organs that the body has. It is even used as an overflow route if other methods of elimination fail. Elimination is vital for health - imagine how quickly a car would react if its exhaust pipe was blocked. If one of more of your body's elimination routes isn't working properly, you get a build-up of waste products that can make you feel dreadful at best, suicidal at worst. It can also put strain on other elimination organs (particularly the liver and kidneys), which have to pick up the slack.

The skin receives a third of all the blood that is circulating around the body. That's why it is quick to react when there's a problem inside the body - it's often one of the first signs that there's an imbalance somewhere.

## THE VITAMIN D BENEFIT

Some Vitamin D is produced via the action of sunlight on the skin - well, it is by skin that isn't clogged and congested anyway! – converting cholesterol in the skin into vitamin D. Proof that not all cholesterol is bad for us!

The symptoms of vitamin D deficiency are varied but can include: bone pain (painful to the touch), muscle weakness, scalp pain, general aches & pains, low mood, fatigue, muscle cramps. In really severe cases, very low vitamin D can even affect the heart.

If you live in a part of the world that gets very little sunlight in winter, skin brushing before a daily walk or sit outside at lunchtime can really help. Rickets (bow legs) is the most widely known problem caused by lack of vitamin D but it was thought to have been eliminated in the 20th century. However it is now reappearing in multiple countries. One reason is people's fear of sunburn, with devoted parents slathering their children in total sun block all summer.

It's a good idea to get 10 minutes of unprotected sun daily to guard against vitamin D deficiency, as well as eating foods that contain the vitamin (although we get most of our vitamin D from the sun) such as eggs and oily fish.

# A NATURAL DETOX & GLOW

Brushing allows the skin to do its part in your body's detoxing. The skin removes about a quarter of the total toxins that the body gets rid of all the time. If the skin is clogged with dead cells it is unable to get rid of that quarter of toxins that it is responsible for, and they go back into the circulation.

Skin brushing not only removes the dead layers of skin, it also keeps pores open and functioning well. It makes your skin better able to do its job of eliminating wastes and toxins.

This also gives the complexion a healthier appearance by removing the things that dull it, improving circulation, and reducing any sagginess.

Not only will your skin be brighter (due to not being clogged with dead skin cells), it will be healthier, softer and more glowing because it will be able to 'breathe'. Cell renewal will have been stimulated and the exchange of wastes and nutrients will have improved. The skin should feel slightly tighter if it was a bit saggy before.

# THE LYMPHATIC SYSTEM

Unless you are medically or anatomically trained, you probably don't give an awful lot of thought to your lymphatic system (maybe even if you *are* medically/anatomically trained!). The only time you think about your lymphatics is when something goes wrong.

I did when I got badly swollen glands under my arms. People who have had lymph glands removed due to cancer certainly think about them. If you have had lymph glands removed from under your arms, your arms can swell up painfully. Those little glands do a great job of filtering out waste products from the body, such as bacteria and fungus.

You probably won't realize that your lymph system has been a little sluggish until you start skin brushing - and that, hopefully, will only be because you start feeling the beneficial effects. You could feel less 'Meh', less sluggish, less toxic. You could feel a renewed energy, a bit of a spring in your step. If you do it properly!

Skin brushing's effect on the lymphatics is one of the most important reasons for taking up the habit. We can stimulate our blood circulation with exercise but lymphatics can be harder to get going, especially if we have health problems.

# THE IMMUNE SYSTEM

If you get regular colds, coughs and sinus infections you may be pleasantly surprised by this benefit. It is because the bacteria and wastes that the lymphatic system transport around the body are dealt with more quickly - they are killed off, moved out, and are not allowed to build up and take over.

When I was ill with CFS I used to get every cold going, one after the other. Since doing daily skin brushing I haven't had a bad one for 9 months, even when people close to me have had them. Skin brushing devotees often report much shorter colds, if they succumb at all.

## THE ENDOCRINE SYSTEM (HORMONES)

Skin brushing stimulates the hormone producing glands. Hormones are produced by the endocrine system, which then releases them into the blood. Ladies, this is a huge one for us. Hormones, far from being the bane of our lives, are the things that make us feminine, that make us feel good and give us our 'get up and go'.

When you start menstruating you can see it as a curse and when you start going through menopause you can see it as another curse. But we should be embracing our hormones. We need them. We only tend to realize that when they start to drop off after menopause and we rush to a doctor to plead for hormone replacement therapy.

Stimulate your body's natural hormone producing glands gently with skin brushing and you can get things going that have been dormant for a while. You can even improve pre-menstrual and menopausal symptoms.

## BLOOD CIRCULATION

Skin brushing increases the blood circulation to the skin. If you accidentally hurt yourself, it is instinctive to rub the area. Why? Because that brings fresh blood to the injury - increasing local circulation - to help heal it with platelets, nutrients, and oxygen.

When we brush our skin we are doing that all over, bringing fresh blood that's full of life-giving oxygen and nutrients.

It gives you a zingy, energetic feeling even if you usually have the get up and go of a chronically depressed sloth.

## MUSCLE TONE

One of the main reasons that I'm willing to strip off in the cold British winter and do an all-over skin brushing routine is because of the massive effect that skin brushing has on muscle tone.

Even without dieting or exercise, you will see an improvement in your body's appearance within a few *days* of starting to do skin brushing.

The reason is that the brushing stimulates the nerve endings in the skin, which activate muscles. It is said that 5 minutes skin brushing is equivalent to 30 minutes jogging in terms of body toning. I've never jogged so I wouldn't be able to confirm that but I was very pleasantly surprised at the improvement in my muscles after just a couple of days of twice daily skin brushing.

My muscles had been quite floppy, due to lack of exercise. My arms weren't too bad as I had been able to do some light weight lifting, even with painful ankles (sitting down), but my thighs were a sorry state as I hadn't been able to do any walking or cycling for years. Now they look like I do exercise!

## CELLULITE

If you don't have cellulite you may want to consider buying a ticket for a lottery occasionally, as you're obviously extremely lucky. Even the most well-toned, hyper-fit people can find the odd bit. It's the dimpled, bubbly skin effect that appears on fatty areas of the body such as the outer thighs and buttocks. Some people compare it to orange peel, but that's doing oranges an injustice.

Most people learn to live with it but others spend a lot of money on creams, lotions, massage devices, and therapies such as ultrasound and electric stimulation. Yet a week or two of daily skin brushing will have an effect on even stubborn cellulite. I think it's a better and longer-lasting effect than most anti-cellulite systems produce, because it is stimulating the body to get rid of the cellulite itself.

Cellulite improves, or disappears, because of the toning effect that skin brushing has on the muscles under the skin, and due to improvement in the lymphatic system.

Try it and see. It will take a couple of months to get rid of the worst cases but most people will see a big improvement after just two weeks. The benefits of dry skin brushing last, in terms of cellulite. I can forget for a few days and my upper arms, which used to be dimply, will still be smooth. I don't know how long you could not do skin brushing and expect cellulite to stay away... because I don't want to try it to find out!

## FATTY DEPOSITS

Fatty deposits are similar to cellulite but can occur anywhere, whereas cellulite generally tends to be restricted to the thighs, buttocks, and upper arms generally. When you put on weight, your existing fat cells swell to store more fat and new fat cells are made. When you lose weight - which is done through eating slightly less than you need so the body has to draw on its fat reserves for energy - the fat cells shrink. Start brushing the skin above them and they can be redistributed so the skin is smooth again.

## DIGESTION/NUTRIENT ABSORPTION

This was a biggie for me. Digestion often slows down when you aren't very mobile. Mine almost stopped. When you get a slow digestive system you often get constipation and it can be painful, uncomfortable, unsocial(!), and extremely energy-sapping. The technique for brushing the abdomen is different to the rest of the body and you have to get it right for brushing to help digestion, but it does help, considerably.

## FLEXIBILITY

This is an often overlooked benefit of skin brushing but it is an important one. When brushing, you have to bend and twist to reach bits of you that you may not have seen for a while. It's movement that we don't otherwise do and it can help with flexibility and stretching.

I noticed an improvement in my Pilates moves after taking up skin brushing, and it was due to the bending and twisting I did every morning and evening with my brush!

## ENERGY

Not when you first drag yourself out of bed - later, after you do your skin brushing routine. There's nothing like it for giving you a bit of zip. Having more energy - especially when you are not used to having any to spare - makes you more likely to make better health choices. It's like cleaning your teeth, you don't tend to want to eat immediately after cleaning your teeth because they feel all smooth and minty. Brush your skin and it's similar. You don't want to stuff your body with rubbish.

# VARICOSE VEINS

Varicose veins are the scourge of those who have to stand for a living. They happen when the little valves inside veins, that prevent a backward flow of blood, get overwhelmed and stop working properly. They swell, blood is allowed to flow backwards and the result is a knotted mess that can be visible through the skin.

You shouldn't EVER brush over varicose veins - that's really important. Those veins are struggling and you don't want to add to their burden by aggravating them. Plus, it could really hurt. But you can brush above and below them (staying well away from the swollen bits) and that will help blood flow and muscle tone and get things moving.

There are other things you can do too. I had varicose veins both times when I was pregnant. The only thing that helped the 'dragging' ache was to lie with my legs up a wall. It lets gravity help the blood flow and allows the valves to drain in the right direction (back towards the heart).

ଓଛଠ

So lots of great reasons to take up skin brushing.

Because of its importance, let's take a deeper look at the lymphatic system and why its health is so vital to our general wellbeing...

# CHAPTER 4
## UNDERSTANDING THE LYMPHATIC SYSTEM

ఆక్షో

BOOKS AND ARTICLES about lymph often annoy me because they almost always start by saying, 'Unlike the blood circulatory system, the lymphatic system has no pump.' Of course it doesn't, you only have one heart! (I wonder if Dr Who's second heart is to pump his lymph – maybe that's why he lives so long!) Other things are too deep, which leave me drifting off mentally and wondering what to cook for dinner in the middle of trying to read some tedious scientific paper.

Just after I started reading about the lymphatic system, I tripped when stepping out of the French doors at my parents' house. It was summer and I had popped inside to get some sun lotion. My foot caught as I was heading back out and I fell onto the deck outside. A white fluid oozed from under me as my mother rushed to pick me up.

I cried, "Oh no! My lymph is leaking!"

It was the sun lotion. I had fallen on the bottle and cracked it. I was fine. My pride, however, was not as my Dad produced an encyclopedia so he could intelligently explain the differences between lymphatic fluid and sun lotion to me. It turns out they're quite different!

Stick with me here. It's a bit heavy but if you persevere you'll get it and it is important to understand a bit about lymph in order to understand why skin brushing works. I love the way the National Library of Medicine defines the function of the lymphatic system:

> *'The lymphatic system is a network of tissues and organs. It is made up mainly of lymph vessels, lymph nodes [glands] and lymph. Lymph filters fluid from around cells. It is an important part of the immune system.*
>
> *When people refer to swollen glands in the neck, they are usually referring to swollen lymph nodes.*
>
> *Common areas where lymph nodes can be easily felt, especially if they are enlarged, are: the groin, armpits (axilla), above the clavicle (supraclavicular), in the neck (cervical), and the back of the head just above the hairline (occipital).'*

## LYMPH'S CONNECTION WITH BLOOD CIRCULATION

The blood circulation transports oxygen, nutrients, and other goodies to the cells all over the body via arteries (which take blood from the heart). The network of blood vessels gets progressively smaller, from the large arteries and veins down to tiny capillaries. The arteries are [mostly[4]] responsible from taking freshly-oxygenated blood away from the heart, and the veins are responsible for taking the blood and wastes back.

Before that, an exchange happens in the capillaries - an exchange of oxygen, CO2, cellular debris, toxins, etc., are picked up and transported in the blood back to the heart.

So arteries bring blood and oxygen to the tissues and veins take blood and wastes away. 90% of what goes into the capillary bed goes back, the other 10% becomes the responsibility of the lymphatic system (which is actually part of the circulatory system).

## THE INTERSTITIAL FLUID (ISF)

Lymphatic fluid is made in the watery part of our bodies, the stuff that we're supposedly 70% made of, called the interstitial fluid (ISF). It is said that if your lymphatic system broke down you would be dead within 24-48 hours.

ISF lives between the cells. It is where the waste products from the blood and the cells end up, together with some water. There is a continual exchange between the blood and the ISF due to different pressures inside and outside the capillaries.

ISF is made at the parts of the capillaries that arterial blood goes into (blood coming from the heart), at the other end, where venous blood is returning blood to the heart, lymph is formed, heading for the lymph capillaries. Lymph is a clear liquid, almost like water and wholly unlike most sun lotions! It is made up of

---

[4] The pulmonary artery and umbilical arteries are the only exceptions to this – they carry deoxygenated blood.

water, dead cells (they have to go somewhere), cell fragments, protein molecules, and fats.

The initial lymph vessels open up to allow the ISF to enter. They are stimulated to open up either by a buildup of fluid/pressure within the interstitial space or when connected skin is stretched. The initial lymph vessels are held in place by collagen and elastin fibers. When the skin is stretched, the elastin fibers are moved, and so is the initial lymphatic vessel, opening it up. So the ISF becomes lymph once it enters the lymphatic system.

> **The initial lymph vessels are stimulated to open up when the skin is STRETCHED.**
> **This bit is important – we can stimulate the delicate initial lymph vessels to open up by skin brushing.**
>
> **Not by vigorous massage, not by trying to force them to open, but by gentle skin brushing with a good brush.**

As the new lymph travels around the lymph channels, it comes into contact with blood and picks up the stuff that needs to be dealt with by the lymph glands or glands (where they beat up the bacteria, pathogens and other toxins, and purify the lymph) and transporting things to other parts of the body.

One of the things the lymphatic system deals with is excess protein. Protein molecules attract water to themselves, so cause swelling. They are also large - too large to get back into the blood stream via the capillaries. The initial lymphatic openings are bigger than the capillaries so are able to deal with troublesome proteins.

Other things the lymphatic system deals with are: dead cells, bacterias, viruses, fats, water, waste products, and inorganic substances.

Some lymph goes back into the bloodstream (to replace volume lost when it was changed into ISF) via the venus (veins) system.

## HOW LYMPH MOVES

Like the veins, the lymph vessels also have one-way valves that encourage the lymph to move in a one-way system.

Some lymphatic vessels have smooth muscle surrounding them. The muscle have stretch sensors. When a sensor stretches, filling up with lymph, it sends a message to the muscle to tell it to contract. This pushes the lymph along.

When the lymph moves away it creates a vacuum, pulling ISF into the initial lymphatic vessel.

So lymph is mainly propelled by peristalsis - the movement of smooth muscle. Peristalsis is also what moves food through the bowels. If your smooth muscle isn't very active, your lymphatic system can be really quite slow. That means not enough lymph is made, not enough converts back into blood, and it doesn't transport the waste products around your body quickly enough or beat up enough of the bad guys in its glands.

The result is you start to feel a bit off color.

If you have had lymph glands removed, aren't very active, and are dealing with the after-effects of chemotherapy, feeling off color is putting it rather too mildly. You feel ghastly.

You can feel almost as ghastly without suffering from cancer though. Anyone who has been immobile for a while finds that their whole body feels sluggish - from their circulation to their digestion. Their skin will look dull and gray, their hair will start to lose its gloss, and they will either crave foods (their body's attempts to get more nutrients) or go off their food (their body's attempts to shed some of its burden, like a hot air balloon that's losing height).

There are a few things that encourage lymph flow, including:

➢ Skeletal muscle contractions - from walking, housework, exercising, etc. These can be from passive exercise as well, including massage or using a machine that moves your body for you, such as a chi machine.

➢ Breathing - deep breathing has a very beneficial effect on the lymphatic system. In fact, MLD therapists usually teach deep breathing to their patients as MLD alone isn't nearly as effective as MLD accompanied by deep breathing.

➢ Pulsing of the arteries - again, encouraged by exercise and deep breathing.

➢ MLD - manual lymphatic drainage activates the stretch response in the lymphatic vessels. This increases the rate of flow of the lymph.

## WHAT DO LYMPH VESSELS LOOK LIKE?

Lymph vessels vary in size but act like a mesh, covering the entire body and surrounding each organ. Some - the initial lymphatics - lie immediately under the surface of the skin. They are held up by collagen and elastin fibbers to keep them in place. These aren't long like pipes, they stand up and look a little like a rubber glove with the fingers pointing upwards towards the skin. These are tiny, fragile vessels - their walls are only one cell thick.

This is why MLD therapists use such gentle movements. They want to stimulate the lymph vessels, not crush them.

## WHAT DO LYMPH GLANDS LOOK LIKE?

Lymph glands are also known as nodes. All lymph vessels lead to lymph glands. They are small oval things, about 1-2cm long, that look a bit like peanuts, although some can be larger. There are between 400 and 700 lymph glands in the body.

They live in clusters at various parts of the lymph system, linked by the lymph vessels. They have a number of functions, including:

- ➢ They act as filters for foreign invaders. Their insides look like honeycombs, so they neatly trap things that shouldn't be there - including cancer cells.
- ➢ They purify the lymph.
- ➢ They produce lymphocytes, which destroy foreign invaders.
- ➢ They contain white blood cells, which fight invaders.

Most people think lymph glands are only found in the clusters that we know of, in the armpit, chest, and neck. But, in fact, half of the glands are found in the abdomen and they are also found throughout the lymphatic system, with larger clusters in the areas we know about.

My Dad had a battle with bowel cancer (he won) and had to have some of the lymph glands nearby removed when he had part of his bowel taken away. He didn't suffer any ill-effects of this. I thought he might get some lymphodema but he didn't, presumably because the lymph easily re-routed.

Breast cancer patients seem to suffer from lymphodema more than any other cancer patients. That's probably because lymph glands are taken from the armpits, causing the arms to swell with excess fluid – almost like it is caught in a traffic jam.

An MLD therapist can not only ease the congestion and reduce the pain of lymphodema, they can also teach the lymph other ways around, avoiding the problem area.

---

You can find an MLD therapist via the
Dr Vodder website or try one of the
cancer charities in your own country.

**www.vodderschool.com/find_a_therapist**

---

The lymph glands absorb a lot of the liquid content of the lymph - around 40%. This has the effect of making the lymph much thicker, because the glands have taken the water.

The lymph glands are therefore the biggest problem in the flow of lymph! Let's take a closer look at where they lie in the body.

# THE MAIN LYMPH CLUSTERS

Whenever we brush we're going to be brushing towards the nearest collection of lymph glands so it's good to know where they are.

### Head & Neck

These are called the cervical lymph glands (cervical means 'relating to the neck') and are mainly towards the outsides of the head – so the cheeks rather than the nose – under the jaw and at the base of the outside of the neck.

### Thorax (the chest & lungs)

This area is often overlooked, or at least under emphasized, by skin brushers but it's very important.

Look at the diagram – there are lots of glands running up the center of the body, as well as towards the sides.

### Abdomen

There are huge collections of lymph glands in the abdomen. They are mainly concentrated slightly out towards the sides, away from the center of the trunk.

### Arms

There are big clusters of glands deep in the armpit and superficially over the shoulder and outer chest, and above the inner elbow.

It's important to brush towards the armpit, as well as up and over the top of the arm, over the shoulder.

### Legs

There are superficial and deep inguinal (groin), and popliteal (back of the knee).

We're going to be brushing towards these lymph gland clusters, to encourage the flow of lymph towards them to be processed (filtered, cleaned up, and moved on) and then onwards back to the circulatory system.

So that's a whistle-stop tour of the lymphatics. When your lymphatics fail, the rest of the body soon fails. So if you get any swelling or tenderness it's time to:

➢ See a doctor. It could be a minor infection or something that needs more investigation;

➢ Reduce stress and take extra care of yourself;

➢ Rehydrate yourself and take some gentle exercise if you are able to;

➢ See a manual lymphatic drainage therapist if you have a chronic problem.

One of the things you can do to stimulate your lymphatic system, other than skin brushing, is rebounding. That's exercise on a mini trampoline. It's unique because it uses gravity to exercise every single cell in the body and it's amazing at getting lymph moving. More on rebounding later on in the book.

Let's look next at whether detoxing – or, rather, helping the body's own natural detoxification systems - is really necessary, as the lymphatic system seems so capable of getting rid of junk all by itself...

# CHAPTER 5
# IS DETOXING NECESSARY?

ෆ৪৯

WHEN NON HEALTH-oriented doctors and nutritionists say that detox diets are pointless due to the incredible power of the body's own detoxification systems they are technically correct. In a healthy, active person with no underlying health problems, there is generally no need to assist the natural detox systems. But there *is* in a non-healthy, non-active person.

Consider what happened to me. I had been very active and healthy. Then I spent weeks in hospital, immobile, after my car wreck and spent years having operations which caused further immobility and required my body to deal with and process lots of anesthetics, painkillers, anti-inflammatories, and other drugs. Moving that lot out of my system was quite a hard job for my body, which was already under stress. Being immobile meant that my muscles weren't doing their job of stimulating the lymphatic system, so I got more and more sluggish.

My case was extreme though. People get sluggish lymph from regular lifestyles - perhaps a job that involves sitting or standing, a diet that includes clogging foods such as cheese and white flour products, from having to take prescription drugs. It can be from poor posture and/or depression or chronic negative thinking (which causes poor posture). It can be from not drinking enough water. The lymphatic system is healthier when the hydration level of the body is good and other organs and systems use a lot of water too.

It has always confused me that doctors understand lymphedema and other illnesses caused by a build-up of toxins - yet they deny the existence of toxins or that there is any need to help the body detoxify, ever!

It seems that you don't have to have had something as serious as cancer and chemotherapy treatment for your natural detoxification systems to be under extreme stress. Of the people I know personally and virtually, so many of them have experienced vast improvements in their health through skin brushing that it seems that their body's detoxing ability had previously been impaired and the skin brushing helped tremendously.

## WHERE DETOXES HAVE FAILED BEFORE

All the detoxes I have seen, tried, or rejected have involved strict regimes of **avoidance**. Often they have good reasons for recommending giving up certain foods, drinks, or habits but giving lots of things up that your body has been relying on is a sure fire way of putting it into a state of stress.

A stressed body is an unhappy body and one that's not willing to let go of its precious stores of fat, especially if it isn't getting enough calories. It's probably spent a long time carefully setting up those fat stores. Imagine taking away a squirrel's hard-earned store of nuts? You'd be in for a pretty serious scratching!

As we saw in the Minnesota Starvation Experiment, the body needs a certain amount of calories and nutrients. Not getting them brings a whole host of unpleasant side-effects (apathy, depression, sensitivity to noise, increased neuroticism, increased preoccupation with food, heightened craving for food, reduction of humor, etc.,). These aren't things that are going to help you stick to a diet, summon up the energy to exercise, or maintain your motivation when things get tough.

Add to that the combination of withdrawal symptoms that you get from giving up caffeine, sugar, alcohol, and other addictive substances. You feel pretty rough and your body becomes convinced there's a war on and it should stuff as much as possible into your fat cells in case famine accompanies the war.

That's why traditional dietary detoxes have failed in the past for many people. That's why I haven't advised giving up any foods or drinks. All I do is advise you to rehydrate by taking in a little more water (if you haven't been drinking much) and adding some things to it to increase your intake of potassium. That's it.

Nourishing your body through skin brushing, gently stimulating your blood and lymph circulation, and rehydrating, are enough to be getting on with. Once you start feeling better, you will find that you won't be craving the foods that you know don't suit you (and that will be individual for you). You'll find that the skin brushing will give you more energy and you'll feel like doing some exercise, or finding some way of moving your body that you're comfortable with.

## DON'T RUSH IN

If your lymph is sluggish and not doing its job properly you don't want to suddenly get it going – and certainly not without ensuring that you're adequately hydrated first. Why? Because it will feel like the worst hangover in living history. You would willingly submit to being guillotined just to get rid of the headache that it can cause.

So when people say the human body doesn't need any help in detoxifying and detox diets and treatments are quackery, I usually put my arms by my sides (I can now the lymph glands in my armpits are no longer swollen and horribly painful), smile, and hope that they never have to find out for themselves that sometimes the body does need some help detoxing.

Dry skin brushing is one of the easiest, cheapest and most effective methods of stimulating your lymphatic system. But before you rush off to find a yard brush and start manically scrubbing your body, let's look at some of the side-effects that can happen if you go at this too quickly...

---

### DETOX RECAP

The body relies on the lymphatic system to process by-products of its detoxification activities. Movement is essential to keep the lymph flowing as it is stimulated by muscle contractions. Skin brushing stimulates lymph, tones up muscles, and improves blood circulation.

If your lymph has been sluggish for a while you will have a buildup of cellular debris, broken-down bacterias, inactivated viruses, etc., clogging up your system.

Take skin brushing *slowly* or you will have such a rush of these flowing around that you'll feel dreadful.

# CHAPTER 6
# THE SIDE-EFFECTS OF RUSHING INTO SKIN BRUSHING

CR80

KARL HERXHEIMER WAS born into a German-Jewish family nearly 20 years after his brother Salomon and probably became such a success in the profession they both shared - dermatology - because he spent his life trying to keep up with the brother who was always 20 years ahead of him. Karl received his doctorate at the tender age of 24 and the brothers worked together.

Karl later became a director of a dermatology clinic with Paul Ehrlich. He and Ehrlich later helped found the University of Frankfurt, where Karl became professor for skin and venereal diseases. He made brilliant discoveries and breakthroughs throughout his career and eventually retired for a well-earned rest.

That ended when he was murdered at the age of 81 by the Nazis at Theresienstadt, the same concentration camp where Sigmund Freud's sister Esther's life was also taken from her.

One of Karl's discoveries was what has become popularly known as the Herxheimer Reaction (or Herxheimer Response) but it's full title is actually the Jarisch-Herxheimer Reaction, as he discovered it with Adolph Jarisch, an Austrian dermatologist. Whether the full name was reduced because Herxheimer is easier to say than Jarisch-Herxheimer, or whether it was because of an understandable wish after World War II to avoid any remembrance of Adolph Hitler is not known.

## THE HERXHEIMER REACTION

Herxheimer and Jarisch noticed that when treating patients who were suffering from syphilis with drugs that killed the syphilis (the treatment then was mercury but antibiotics were used later), they got temporarily worse. Their symptoms increased even though the syphilis was dying. The reaction was an inflammatory one (increased inflammatory cytokines were found) and was seen in between 50 & 90% of patients.

Naturopaths have taken the Herxheimer Reaction name to apply to what happens when a disease or other problem is treated and the effects of the disease dying cause additional symptoms. What naturopaths mean today by a Herxheimer Reaction isn't exactly the same as the original Herxheimer Reaction but it is now meant to mean the body's response to the curing of a disease or disorder, when that response causes unpleasant symptoms in the patient. It's also called a Healing Crisis. That's a good name too, because it does feel like a crisis when you're going through it.

It's pretty easy to understand when you think of it this way: If you had a big, bad bacterial disease, that would be because bacteria had invaded your body and overwhelmed the good guys in your immune system. The bacteria had multiplied and you had developed all sorts of horrible symptoms. Suppose I came along with a wonderful new antibiotic that promised to kill all the bad bacteria really, really quickly. You'd probably be delighted and guzzle it gleefully. Until the bacteria started being killed. As they died, like all organisms, they would start breaking down. Think of a banana left on a sunny window ledge for a week or so. It goes brown, then starts stinking and turning into gooey slime. That's what would happen to the dying and dead bacteria in your body. As they broke down, they would start to release toxins - a lot of toxins - which your body would have to deal with. Depending on the health of your body, this could take a short time (just a few hours) or a long time (several days or weeks) to deal with.

You would react to the toxins in a way totally individual to your make-up, it could be severe headaches, joint or muscle pains, inability to think clearly, fever, fast heartbeat, and many more. Each person's body comes up with novel ways of reacting to these things!

It also depends on the length of time you have been ill and the severity of your illness (how many bad guys have been allowed to establish a presence and how deeply entrenched they have become - i.e. whether they are still camping in tents or have established permanent homes with foundations and extensions).

Then you would react to your body's attempts to deal with the disposal of the bad guys' remains and the release of the toxins from their breaking-down forms. Your body would get very, very busy inside. It would be making new white blood cells, transport the toxins to safe areas, send them into the lymph, where the glands would deal with them and break them down further. There would be a lot going on. As this is essential work, your body wouldn't be worried about you feeling a little under the weather. It wouldn't have the resources to spare to deal with your piddling little complaints, it would be too busy!

That's the modern Herxheimer Reaction. It's a reaction to being cured. A reaction to the release of toxins from the breaking down of the things that caused your illness in the first place.

That illness could be one or many. It could be something recognized by doctors because it has been reported enough times to appear in their medical books. Or it could be something that hasn't been officially recognized but is no less debilitating and energy-sapping.

A modern Herxheimer Reaction can also be known as a cleansing crisis, cleaning reaction, or healing crisis.

## DON'T ASSUME YOU ARE HAVING A HERXHEIMER-TYPE REACTION

A young man who featured in a TV documentary 30-odd years ago thought he was just going through an extended cleansing crisis, or Herxheimer Reaction.

He was little more than a creaking skeleton. There were deep circles under his hollow eyes and he moved his wasted limbs carefully, clearly in pain. Yet when he spoke there was hope in his voice. He didn't focus on his illness, but spoke about journaling his journey of recovery. All he wanted was to help others, to make some sense of his own suffering. He was convinced that the health regime he had embarked on would heal his body and enable him to teach others how to do the same.

I wish I could remember his name, or at least the name of the TV program that featured his story. He deserves to be remembered as more than a victim of AIDS. His beautiful soul shone through, despite his ravaged body.

The last months of that young man's life were spent in needless pain. There were drugs to help, even back then. But he was determined to stick to a punishing detox 'health' regimen, convinced that what he was suffering was just a Herxheimer Reaction and the regimen would enable his broken immune system to fight back.

That's why detox diets **can** be dangerous. That's why when you read a disclaimer on a health book, diet, or supplement, advising you to consult your doctor before starting, then you really should, and not put any symptoms down to diet, cleansing, or supplements. I know that doctors often don't seem remotely interested when you mention these things but it could be that they put you on some blood pressure medication recently and need to remind you not to eat grapefruit on your new diet (which can negatively interact with a number of drugs). Perhaps you suddenly start suffering from headaches when you start skin brushing - it is dangerous to assume that they are just the result of the skin brushing, get checked out.

Doctors have seen things that the rest of us haven't. They have seen the results of interactions from innocent-sounding supplements and the results of people trying to self-medicate.

I suffered a drug reaction myself. I was taking a natural supplement, tryptophan (an amino acid) from a health food store to help depression, at the same time as a prescribed antihistamine for summer allergies. I didn't realize that my daily, ever worsening headaches could be anything to do with these simple tablets. I put it down to posture - assuming I must have been hunching over my computer – so kept downing painkillers, while attempting to sit properly. It was the interaction of tryptophan and the antihistamine. The headaches stopped within 24-hours when I stopped taking them.

Sometimes doctors do know best. Get any new symptoms checked.

## HOW TO AVOID A HERXHEIMER/CLEANSING REACTION

Please believe me when I say that you don't ever want to experience a full-blown Herxheimer/cleansing reaction. It's not just unpleasant, it feels like you're dying. If you regularly drink coffee or another high-caffeine drink, and have ever had to go without it for a day or two, you will know what a caffeine withdrawal headache is like. It's awful. Multiply that by about 100 and you'll have some idea what a bad Herxheimer/cleansing reaction is like.

Now if you are crazy enough to do what I did and suddenly adopt a 'clean', healthy lifestyle after having had 'bad', unhealthy habits for some time, you will go through a Herxheimer/cleansing reaction - especially if you include dry skin brushing in your routine. That's because the brushing stimulates the lymph when it is busy processing all the toxins that are being dumped in its little detoxifying plants (the glands), and it ends up sending some of the toxins out unprocessed. So you get toxins circulating around your body, leaving you feeling rough.

You can do a few things to avoid a bad reaction:

> Monitor your urine output to see if you need to increase you water intake. If your urine is very pale you're fine but if it is yellow or darker (and you haven't been taking B

vitamins, which can cause it to go fluorescent!) then you should increase the amount of water that you drink. Start with having a glass soon after you wake up and one before bed. Sip some more throughout the day until your urine is almost clear.

➤ Eat more potassium-rich foods (green vegetables, lentils, sweet potatoes, white beans).

➤ Eat more water-rich foods (fruits and vegetables).

➤ Start skin brushing slowly at first.

➤ Get some sunshine, if possible.

➤ Do some light non-stressy exercise - such as gentle swimming, Pilates, or yoga.

➤ Try some rebounding (more on that later).

➤ Take some vitamin C or [preferably] add freshly squeezed lemon juice to your water.

➤ Do some deep breathing.

➤ Don't do anything else! In particular, don't give up any foods or drinks that you usually have, don't suddenly take up running, don't even stop drinking alcohol if you usually partake regularly.

We're going to start by increasing your water intake, then begin skin brushing gently, gradually, so your body has time to adapt and get used to it.

Remember that while the syphilis patients in Herxheimer's original studies didn't all experience the reaction, between 50 and 90% of them did. Some may not have had the disease for long, others may have been fitter and healthier generally or had strong immune and lymphatic systems.

If you do experience what you believe to be a Herxheimer/cleansing reaction, get your doctor's opinion, don't assume.

Next, let's look at what you need – if you don't already have one – a brush …

# Chapter 7
# Order Your Brush

❦

I LOVE BAMBOO brushes with vegetable fibers. They are available from health food stores and online suppliers such as Amazon. They are firm enough to move your skin when you brush but soft enough not to scratch or irritate. Brushes with natural bristles made from plant fibers are the best - they are generally made for skin brushing. Look for ones labeled as being for skin brushing or dry skin brushing.

If you can find a good natural brush close to home, go ahead and buy one. Just make sure it is firm enough. It needs to feel really quite firm, nothing like regular bath brushes, which tend to be too soft. You need one that is a little more like a vegetable scrubbing brush!

If you buy a stiff brush, you can brush lightly to get a lighter effect but if you have a soft and floppy brush you can't alter the pressure to get a more vigorous, energizing brushing because the bristles will just flop over.

The bristles should bend only slightly when you brush firmly against your skin. Test it on the back of your hand (lightly) to make sure that it is firm but doesn't scratch. Scratchy bristles are not helpful for skin brushing. If you rub the brush across the top of your hand, firmly, it shouldn't leave any marks or indentations.

Don't panic and think you'll never get used to such a stiff brush. Most people report that their brush felt very firm for the first two or three uses but then they got used to it and it felt 'normal'. That was my experience as well.

I love the Bernard Jensen skin brush that Amazon.com generally has in stock.

### http://amzn.com/B0016BM5D2

Expect to pay $10-15 for your brush - the Bernard Jensen one I mentioned is $12. A good one will last many years, with care.

Which leads us to...

## BRUSH CARE

Brushes don't need a lot of pampering but there are a few things you can do to prolong the life of your brush, keep it working hard for you, and ensure that you are getting the best effects from it.

When you first start skin brushing it is best to wash your brush after the first week. That's because you will be removing quite a build-up of dead skin cells, which could clog your brush. After a week of brushing you will have removed all the older dead cells and your brush won't need washing very often. Go by its appearance and smell. You can get away with not washing a brush for quite a long time! The more you wash your brush, the more you reduce its lifespan and stiffness. No big deal if you don't mind replacing it every couple of years but if cost is an issue then only use it on freshly washed skin, keep it in a clean place, and don't wash it very often.

Here's how to wash it:

> ➢ Fill the sink or bowel with warm (not hot) water. Squeeze in a squirt of gentle shampoo and swish to make bubbles.

> ➢ Remove the handle from your brush and put the brush into the sink. Swish it around underwater for a few seconds.

> ➢ Remove the brush from the water and hold it over the sink for a few seconds to let the water drip off.

> ➢ Place it on a towel, bristles down, in a warm place. That could be near a window, to use the warmth of the sun, or near a radiator or other gentle heat source. That's **near** a heat source, not **on**, which could warp the brush.

If you don't have a suitable heat source, it will dry anyway on the towel within about 24 hours (depending on your climate).

Many people recommend keeping your brush to yourself for hygienic reasons. That does make sense but I've shared a brush with my daughter when traveling without calamity. We wouldn't share if either of us had any skin problems or abrasions (we probably wouldn't brush with skin problems anyway). We usually wash the brush every other day when sharing.

# HOW OFTEN SHOULD YOU REPLACE YOUR BRUSH?

It depends on the brush's condition. A good brush can last a decade or more. I've had my brush for over 20 years and it's still going strong. For that reason, it is worth buying the best quality brush you can afford, as it will last longer and be better value for money.

You will need to consider replacing your brush when:

- The bristles no longer hold the brush up when placing the brush bristle-down on a table.
- The bristles don't feel firm when pressing the brush against your skin.
- The brush no longer moves the skin but glides over it.
- The bristles start to scratch your skin.
- It gets dirt in it that won't wash out.
- The wood cracks.
- The handle breaks.
- Mold forms on the wood (replace it straightaway).

None of these things have happened to my brush yet so I'm more than happy to keep using it. I would estimate that even an inexpensive brush could be used for two or more years without needing replacing.

It's not a good idea to store your brush in the bathroom, as it could get moldy. A bedroom is better. Mine lives in a drawer where I keep my hairbrush and comb.

While you are waiting for your brush to arrive you can start to learn the skin brushing movements - with your hands...

# PART TWO

---

# THE PLAN

# CHAPTER 8
## WHAT TO DO FIRST

கு8ல

**E**ASY DOES IT. That's good isn't it? It means it's not going to be too difficult!

Don't think about removing things while you are doing this 10-day detox. The introduction of skin brushing will be enough of a shock for your body to be getting on with. Start really taking care of your body for these next ten days, let it know you are batting for it.

These are the steps:

1. Rehydrate – being guided by the color of your 'output' (urine), start drinking a little more water, preferably with some added fresh lemon juice, greens powder[5], or pure cranberry juice.
2. Start doing deep, rhythmic breathing.
3. Start skin brushing – you can start without the brush if you are waiting for your brush to arrive, just use your hands to

---

[5] Powdered vegetables and herbs. Sounds awful but most brands actually taste great.

get used to the movements. For the first few days, just brush each section of your body twice. Once you're used to it, you can increase the number of brush strokes on each section.

That's it. Easy enough to do for 10 days - and, once you have established the habit, simple enough to incorporate into your lifestyle forever. That will bring you long-term benefits.

Later on, you may want to add some extra goodies into your life to nourish your mind and body and help reduce the stress you experience.

If you're ready, let's start the steps...

# CHAPTER 9
## STEP ONE - REHYDRATE

CX8O

MAGAZINES ARE FULL of advice to drink more water but they rarely point out that it is possible to drink too much water. There have been some well publicized deaths due to water intoxication, or hyponatremia.

> DEFINITION: *hyponatremia*
>
> *A condition in which the amount of sodium (salt) in the blood is lower than normal.*
>
> US National Library of Medicine

I've long been interested in this because my body seems to have a bigger need for water than other people's bodies! I know plenty of people who exist on a few cups of tea or coffee a day. If I did that I'd probably pass out. If I don't drink 5 or more glasses of water a day I start to feel a bit ill first and very ill later. Constipation and abdominal gripes are usually the first reminder that I haven't been drinking enough, then my eyes start to look less lively, and my skin more puffy. Finally, dry skin and depression hit (plus back pain if I let the constipation continue). They are certainly strong enough symptoms to make me take notice!

So I was surprised when Dr Eric Berg spoke against the oft-quoted '8 glasses a day' rule. He points out that it is fairly pointless to increase your intake of water unless you increase your intake of potassium, a mineral that works in conjunction with sodium.

Sodium generally lives in the fluids that surround cells – it is important for maintaining blood pressure. We do need sodium, just not too much. Many of us get way too much because we eat processed foods. That throws off the delicate mineral salts balance in our bodies, giving us too much sodium and not enough potassium and other mineral salts (such as calcium, chloride, magnesium, bicarbonate, phosphate, and sulfate).

There is the opposite side of the coin, though, too little sodium. The website MedicineNet quoted a survey[6] of Boston Marathon runners. It revealed that 62 out of 488 runners who gave blood samples had abnormally low sodium levels in their blood. That means they had been sweating a lot (losing sodium) and replacing it with water (without much natural sodium). This is what doctors mean when they talk about electrolyte balance. It's when we lose a lot of the mineral salts from our blood that really need to be there. It can be dangerous, which is why athletes have died from hyponatremia[7].

---

[6] http://bit.ly/bostonhypo

[7] There are many other causes of hyponatremia, including burns, heart failure, cirrhosis, and diarrhea.

That's why they often drink electrolyte drinks, to replace the lost mineral salts. That's also why the rest of us who aren't exercising hard and sweating a lot *shouldn't* be drinking electrolyte drinks, as we can upset the mineral salt balance by doing that.

It's understandable that sweating athletes could be in danger of drinking too much water and upsetting their sodium balance. There is also a danger of drinking too much water when taking some drugs, such as ecstasy. Ecstasy causes a burst of energy, resulting in massive physical activity - often dancing - which in turn causes huge thirst due to sweating.

However, unless you are one of the rare people who habitually drink too much water, you are more likely to be borderline dehydrated. You'd probably know if you had a problem and were drinking water to excess. Excess is likely to involve pints and pints of water at a time.

That's why thinking that you absolutely HAVE to drink 8 glasses of water a day can be harmful. Overriding the body's thirst mechanism isn't a good idea. Convincing yourself that you have to drink 8 glasses no matter what just introduces stress into your life about a perfectly natural thing. It is far better to listen to your body and follow its promptings to drink water.

Diets and articles that tell us to drink when we're not thirsty aren't helpful. They often say that if you are thirsty you're already dehydrated and you should drink before you're thirsty to ensure that you don't get dehydrated. Not helpful. Teaching the body that you're willing to override its promptings could stop it alerting you to possible problems. For example, you don't want it to stop telling you that you've had enough to eat already!

Shockingly, some of Dr Berg's patients who proved to be dehydrated were actually drinking plenty of water. This comes back to the potassium/sodium balance.

Drink a little more water, yes, but also take in **more green vegetables** for the extra potassium and other mineral salts. I say 'take in' for those who don't like eating green vegetables, you can juice them or use greens powder instead.

Doing it this way will help keep your potassium levels high enough for your cells to actually benefit from the water as it will keep the right balance of mineral salts in the fluids in and surrounding the cells.

Low potassium levels are linked to numerous health problems including, according to the Children's National Medical Center in Washington, DC:

> ➤ Lung disorders.
> ➤ Kidney disease.
> ➤ Hypertension.

Other studies have demonstrated potassium's ability to lower high blood pressure[8].

There are foods that actually **deplete** potassium in the body, including:

> ➤ Salty foods - pretzels, crackers, peanuts.
> ➤ Alcoholic drinks.
> ➤ Coffee and sodas.

---

[8] www.naturalnews.com/024539_potassium_sodium_diet.html

So if you eat a lot of salty foods and drink a lot of coffee, sodas, or alcohol, you may want to pay particular attention to your potassium intake.

Many people think that eating a banana gives them all the potassium they need but a banana only contains 422mg of potassium. You would have to eat 10 bananas a day to get all you need as the body needs 4,700 milligrams of potassium. That's a lot of fruit sugar - not ideal.

Getting enough potassium can seem like too much work, so many people resort to potassium supplements or potassium (i.e. reduced sodium) salt. While these can help a little, they aren't great because the potassium they contain isn't as easily absorbable by the body as the potassium from fruits and vegetables.

Potassium supplements should really only be taken on medical advice. Certainly if you have any health problems or take any prescription drugs, don't put yourself on a potassium supplement, get a doctor's approval first.

Increasing your potassium naturally through foods is safer, because you aren't taking the potassium in isolation, it comes with other minerals. It really isn't difficult. Try adding some of the foods on the list below into your usual meals, if they don't already make up part of your diet.

Potassium-rich foods include:

> ➢ White beans (561mg per 100g)
> ➢ Dried coconut (543mg per 100g)
> ➢ Sunflower seeds (645mg per 100g)
> ➢ Lentils - it is easy to eat more lentils. They are high fiber and low fat as well as bursting with potassium. They're a

good source of vegetarian protein too. Add a handful to soups, stews, and casseroles. I like to grind red lentils and add them to bakes as a sort of hamburger helper. (955mg per 100g – or 115mg in just a tablespoon!)

➤ Dark leafy vegetables such as kale, spinach, collard greens. If you don't like them, try them juiced, with vegetables that you do like. Add an apple or carrots to sweeten the juice if you aren't used to green juices. Juices are a great way to get instant liquid nutrition and they don't tax your digestive system so you don't feel tired after drinking them. (558mg per 100g)

➤ Dates. Good on their own or in scones, raw cheesecakes, and raw chocolates. (584mg per 100g)

➤ Sweet potatoes - delicious baked, like standard potatoes. Sweet potatoes are better for blood sugar than standard potatoes. (640mg per 100g - about 15% of your daily requirement.)

➤ Apricots - be careful with dried apricots, they can contain added sugar. There are brands without sugar and preservatives. Prunes and peaches are also good. (1162mg per 100g)

➤ Avocados. If you don't like them, try making raw chocolate, it's wonderful and guilt-free. (485mg per 100g)

➤ Yogurt. (255mg per 100g)

➤ Mushrooms. Easily hidden in casseroles and bakes if you aren't keen on them whole. (396mg per 100g)

➤ Bananas (358mg per 100g)

➤ Tomatoes. Add tomatoes to casseroles, salads, bakes, and anything else you can think of. They are low calorie but packed with potassium, vitamin E, and lycopene. (400mg in 100g of fresh tomatoes. 2455mg in 100g of tomato paste - but you'd probably never eat that much paste!)

Other foods that have good levels of potassium include beans, broccoli, chlorella, dulse, figs, fish, kiwi, mangoes, meat, melons, nuts, oranges, papayas, parsnips, pears, pumpkins, spirulina, squash, yams, zucchini.

## DO I NEED AN ELECTROLYTE DRINK/SUPPLEMENT?

> *"An electrolyte is an electrically-charged mineral like calcium, potassium, magnesium that allows fluid to travel through the body.*
>
> *It allows the nervous system to work, it allows the heart to pump. So we need electrolytes and that's what hydrates us.*
>
> *Water by itself does not hydrate."*
>
> Dr Eric Berg

Electrolyte drinks and 'vitamin' waters are generally made from chemical-based ingredients and usually have large quantities of sugar in them.

We're told to drink electrolyte waters if we suffer from diarrhea or perform athletics in hot weather. They are about the only times we need to. The rest of the time we *can* get all the electrolytes we need from our food. However, people think they need to drink these high sugar/salt combinations if they just go for a stroll on a warm day. They don't!

If you are increasing your water intake you do need to give some consideration to electrolytes, so you don't get your sodium/potassium balance off.

The easiest way is to eat (or drink) more green vegetables. I also use a greens powder, just a teaspoon twice a day and it has made a huge difference to my hydration.

Dr Berg has a recipe for what he calls a weight loss shake on his YouTube channel:

**www.youtube.com/watch?v=TrEPCiihgoQ**

This is a mineral-rich blend of cranberry, lemon or lime, and apple cider vinegar. Something of an acquired taste but a great thing to make up if you have to drink a lot of water, perhaps because of exercise or heat.

The American Heart Association points out on its website (**www.heart.org**) the dangers of too much sodium in terms of high blood pressure and heart problems. The AHA says that potassium is a 'potent weapon' because:

> *The more potassium we consume, the more sodium is excreted through urine and out of the body. Potassium helps relax blood vessel walls, which helps lower blood pressure.*

They also point out that potassium rich foods are more beneficial than potassium-rich salt substitutes, as these can be harmful for certain medical conditions.

## HOW TO TELL IF YOU'RE DEHYDRATED

If you believed the health magazines you could think the most people are walking round like zombies from The Walking Dead, chronically dehydrated and about to collapse. Some people do feel like that but possibly for other reasons!

That said, I do believe that many people suffer from some degree of dehydration. Often they don't realize because they have been dehydrated for most of their adult lives and don't know what it's like to feel hydrated.

I know lots of people who are almost scared to drink more because they don't want to be rushing to the bathroom all the time. That's not a great reason for allowing yourself to get dehydrated, because the effects of dehydration can be quite serious.

Here are a few signs that you may not be sufficiently hydrated:

- Dry or sticky mouth.
- Increased thirst.
- Dry eyes.
- Tiredness.
- Decreased urine output.
- Dark urine.
- Dry skin.
- Headache.
- Dizziness.
- Constipation.
- Lack of sweating.
- Skin doesn't bounce back when pinched slightly.

- ➤ Rapid heartbeat.
- ➤ Rapid breathing.
- ➤ Low blood pressure.
- ➤ Fever.

The Mayo Clinic says that:

> **Thirst isn't always a reliable gauge of the body's need for water, especially in children and older adults.**
>
> **A better indicator is the color of your urine ... dark yellow or amber color usually signals dehydration.**

Good advice. Going on your urine output, rather than a feeling of thirst, works in any climate.

We are so used to not listening to our bodies when they alert us to potential problems that we can override our natural thirst mechanism. Sometimes we will eat instead of drinking. That's why it's a good idea to keep an eye on your urine output. If it looks darker, have a little more water. If it is very pale, ease up on the drinking.

Being properly hydrated (i.e. not too much water, not too little) affects every body system and makes you feel good.

If you have been either drinking too little water or drinking too much, you won't be properly hydrated. Rehydrating your body will help its natural detoxification processes.

# FIRST REHYDRATION HABIT

Start simply by making it a habit to begin each day with a glass of water. Good water if you can - home-filtered or bought spring/mineral water – but in many areas tap water is fine. Try to drink it within an hour of waking up - so it can stimulate your metabolism. Sip it over the course of a few minutes, don't chug it down all at once. You could, if you have time, try drinking it while doing a bit of deep breathing. It's a lovely way to wake your body naturally, instead of leaping/falling out of bed and rushing headlong into the stresses of the day.

If you check your urine first thing in the morning, it will naturally be slightly darker than later in the day, because it is more concentrated for being stored overnight. Check it throughout the day and try to tune into your thirst. You could find that you've been overriding it, either by being too busy, too distracted, or through eating instead of drinking when your body alerts you to the problem.

Have more water throughout the day when you are thirsty and/or when your urine looks dark. Continue to have whatever you normally drink – coffee, tea, sodas, etc., - but have some water as well.

I had a routine blood test recently and the nurse checked with me that I had drunk some water that morning. I asked her why that was important. She explained that veins are very hard to get into with a needle if they aren't properly hydrated. They collapse, there's hardly anything there to get the little needle into. People who are adequately hydrated have beautiful, glossy, squishy veins, she said, that are easy to find and less painful to slip a needle into.

Interesting. So drinking enough water affects much more than we think!

## SECOND REHYDRATION HABIT

Add more mineral salts, especially potassium. Just drinking more water won't hydrate you – you need to increase your intake of potassium. If you can, always add something to your water to add a little potassium.

Try:

> ➢ A squeeze of fresh lemon or lime;
> ➢ A teaspoon of greens powder;
> ➢ Some natural (no sugar) cranberry juice.

Later in the day, have some of the foods from the high potassium list. Here are a few suggestions:

> ➢ A 'slow carb' breakfast of scrambled eggs, spinach, and lentils. This is the breakfast of Tim Ferriss, author of 'The Four Hour Body'. It's packed with protein (to fill you up until lunchtime), vitamins, and minerals, including lots of potassium. Just don't add too much salt! A light sprinkling of a good sea salt blend (I love Vogel's *Herbamare*, which is a brilliant blend of organic herbs, vegetables, and sea salt).
> ➢ A home-made smoothie using a banana, a mango, some sunflower and/or flax seeds, a little yoghurt or milk (I love almond milk) and some coconut or coconut oil. Coconut oil is a terrific thing to add to your diet, being rich in medium-chain fatty acids. You'll find you have more energy and better skin by adding some coconut oil to your diet every day.

> A bowl of yoghurt, topped with a tablespoon of sunflower seeds and a sprinkling of cinnamon. Really delicious. Cinnamon, like coconut, is quite a super food and worth adding to your diet every day. It regulates blood sugar, is warming, and can even help menstrual pain.

> A bowl of yoghurt and desiccated coconut.

> Apricots soaked in milk or yoghurt. Left in the refrigerator for a few hours, the apricots swell and turn into a delicious dessert.

> A salad of mixed leafs and vegetables, including mushrooms, avocados, and/or tomatoes.

> Sweet potato [yam] mash with your dinner.

> If you're okay with gluten, some home-made scones, using wholemeal flour and dates.

That's it. Just paying attention to your urine output, tuning into your thirst mechanism, and possibly having a little more water and some mineral salts via lemon/lime, greens, or cranberry to make sure that it actually rehydrates.

No cutting out other things or you could get side-effects and withdrawal symptoms which could throw you off your skin brushing routine.

## A BIT MORE ABOUT LEMONS

My daughter, reading through the first draft of this book, said, "Have you bought shares in a lemon orchard? You mention them on nearly every page!"

The truth is I love lemons because they are so inexpensive and widely available but they have so many health benefits. And, no, I don't have shares in a lemon orchard!

I usually squeeze a fresh lemon each morning and store it in a little Mason jar in my refrigerator. I just pour a little into a glass of water a couple of times a day. It keeps me feeling fresh and invigorated.

Lemons are packed full of vitamin C and they are anti-bacterial, anti-fungal, and astringent. Almost a superfood, really.

A study into the antimicrobial activity of lemon by the Maxwell Scientific Organization was reported in the British Journal of Pharmacology & Toxicology in March 2011. They used an extract of lemon peel and showed that it is:

> *"Not only an astringent but also*
> *a good antimicrobial agent."*

So if you are concerned about the quality of the water you're drinking – as long as it has actually been declared for human consumption! – then lemon will improve it. City water often tastes bad, that's where lemon comes in very handy.

Lemons also have an alkaline effect on the body when ingested. Most people are shocked at that, because they have a reputation for being acidic... but they aren't in the human body. That's because citric acid, abundant in lemons, is - as acids go - quite weak and is easily processed by the body, which uses it to deal with uric acid (left over when protein is metabolized) then gets rid of it by sweating and breathing it out. Stronger acids are eliminated by urination, which means that they have to be neutralized first, using up some of the body's stores of calcium. As we do a lot of breathing and often a fair bit of sweating, citric acid is easy for the body to handle.

Lemons are alkaline-forming in the body because of their mineral content. They contain calcium as well as other minerals, including magnesium, the all-important potassium, and selenium, meaning that they deal with themselves in the body and don't use up resources.

Then, of course, there's the vitamin C. You would have to eat two lemons to get the vitamin C you would get in an orange but they contain less sugar (less of a glycemic load) so have the edge there. Taking lemon juice in water is a wonderful way of getting an energizing boost of vitamin C.

A squeeze of fresh lemon juice to your morning water will supply you with a good amount of vitamin C and electrolytes, and it will have an alkalizing, cleansing effect on your body. It will even help your immune system deal with invaders and nasties and will stimulate the liver, helping it in its job of being the body's main chemical processing (i.e. detoxification) plant. That's hugely important.

If squeezing a lemon is too much hassle - mornings can be busy - cut a slice off a lemon and pop it into a cup, then pour boiling water over it. There's no need to peel the lemon if it is organic and unwaxed, just give it a good scrub under running water. If it isn't organic/unwaxed, peel the yellow skin off it before slicing it (easy to do with a carrot or potato peeler, which will remove the rind and leave the pith, which is full of nutrients).

# OPTIONAL EXTRAS TO HELP WATER-RESISTANT PEOPLE!

If you don't like the taste - or lack of taste - of water you aren't alone. I know a lot of people who actively dislike water. One of them was my ex mother-in-law. She never drank water. She existed on her beloved coffee. In later life she developed horrible kidney problems, which ended up with her needing regular surgeries. Eventually her whole personality disappeared with the living death of dementia. She had always felt better after her kidney surgeries, as they put her on a drip for a few days. Even the dementia was better after her surgeries.

One of the last images I have of her in my mind was before the dementia got too bad. She was sitting at home, swathed in blankets and jumpers, as it was cold. Her once beautiful skin was shrunken and gray, her eyes sunken, her hands thin and wizened. I'm still wracked with guilt, wishing I had been more vocal in my efforts to get my stubborn ex father-in-law to encourage her to drink some water.

If you don't like water it is vital that you do whatever you have to do make it more palatable so that you will drink more. Here are a few things you can try:

## Fizz It Up

Carbonated water can be bought or made using a Sodastream. A lot of people who don't like plain water will happily drink carbonated water.

Once you're used to drinking more water you may be able to try some without carbonation and wean yourself off it, as it can be bloating.

## Get Clever With Tap Water

Tap water varies in both quality and taste. Some has too much chlorine, which can have an off-putting taste or smell. One trick is to run the tap for a few seconds before letting the water run into your container. Leave the lid off for an hour - which is the time it takes for the chlorine to evaporate. It should taste better. Add some lemon and ice if you need something extra.

Drinking your water from a beautiful glass also makes a difference to how it tastes. I dislike the taste of water from a plastic container but will happily drink the same water from a nice glass. Go figure!

## Try Different Waters

The UK's Queen Elizabeth travels with huge cases of her favorite bottled water, Malvern. Miranda Priestly, the horrendous fashion editor in 'The Devil Wears Prada' only drank San Pellegrino water (but that probably had more to do with product placement!). People have their favorites. Find yours, it can really help. I'm fortunate that I like a relatively inexpensive supermarket brand of bottled water for times when I need to buy some - days out, for example.

## Try Different Temperatures

My son will only drink water if it's ice cold. Fine, throw some ice in. I don't like cold water and don't keep my water filter jug in the refrigerator. Each to their own. Try your water iced or warmed – whatever it takes to get you to drink it.

## Try Adding Things

Freeze some slices of lemon or lime or some berries to add to your water.

Make a pot of your favorite herbal tea, allow it to cool, then pour into ice cube trays and freeze. Add a few cubes to a glass of water.

Make A Vitamin Water. The commercial ones are just sugar and chemicals. Make your own by putting combinations of fruit, vegetables, and herbs in a pitcher and topping up with water. Leave it in the refrigerator for a few hours before drinking. Tasty, nutritious, and delicious. Vitamins are water soluble so they are released into the water. You can even eat the fruit/veg afterwards! Children love these. Here are some good combinations:

> Cucumber & lime.
> Pineapple & mint.
> Lemon & strawberry.
> Apple & cinnamon (use either a teaspoon of ground cinnamon or add a stick to the pitcher). This one is my favorite in winter.

## Drink It Anyway!

Please excuse me, I'm not being cruel, I'm just passionate about health. I can't get over not being able to help my ex mother-in-law and I don't want anyone else to suffer the way she has – for such a simple, easy to fix reason.

If you found out that you had a terrible illness and the only way to cure it was to drink water, you could probably bring yourself to do so, even if you loathe the taste.

Well, drinking water is a way to **avoid** terrible illnesses. It's such a pity that it often takes a crisis to make us do the things that we should have been doing all along. Like when you have an appointment with a dentist – you suddenly start cleaning your teeth really well!

Heart and stroke patients who survive often become healthier than others around them, because they have such a massive incentive to adopt a healthy diet and healthier habits.

If it helps, try imagining you have an expensive appointment with a kidney specialist and start drinking more water so he/she doesn't nag you when they see the color of your urine output!

## ABOUT PLASTIC BOTTLES

There have been rumors circulating about plastic bottles of water. Sheryl Crow stated on the 'Ellen' show that her oncologist told her women should not drink bottled water that has been left in a hot car. Allegedly the oncologist said the heat causes a reaction with chemicals in the plastic, releasing dioxins - which are frequently found in breast cancer tissues. According to the website *Urban Legends*, the FDA has refuted this.

However a European study did find things to be concerned about in plastic bottles. It's probably fine to use plastic bottles occasionally but, whenever you can, choose water in glass bottles and use glass containers at home.

Pretty glass jugs aren't expensive and make plain tap water seem special.

## ABOUT WATER FILTERS

I use a simple jug filter for my water but I am happy to drink tap water in most cities in the west. I simply do a few things to improve the quality and taste:

> ➢ Run the tap for about 30 seconds before pouring any into a glass or jug. New York City department of Environmental Protection even produce a poster for people to download to remind them to do this. Not because the water isn't safe, but because some people have old plumbing in their homes and offices and running the tap for 30 seconds allows any lead that has dissolved into the water (while it was sitting in the faucet) to run off.

> ➢ Leave it standing for a while before drinking it (an hour, ideally, but any length of time gives the chlorine gas some chance to evaporate).

> ➢ Add a slice or squeeze of fresh lemon. Lime will do if you don't have lemon. Artificial lemon isn't effective as it has usually been heat treated and rendered inactive.

There's a lot of anxiety around water. People go to extremes to buy all kinds of filters and purification systems. I'm of the opinion that you do what you can with the resources you have. If you can afford a whole house water purification system, go ahead and get one and enjoy it.

If you can't, don't fret, just do what you can and rest assured that the chorine the water authorities add is there for a very good reason – to kill all kinds of nasty things such as giardia and cryptosporidium.

# CHAPTER 10
## STEP TWO - BREATHING ROUTINE

☙❦❧

THIS ISN'T A chapter to skip over. This is an important part of the plan because it will help support your body's natural detoxification processes, which you are going to be stimulating with the skin brushing in the next step.

It also has some surprising hidden benefits as well. You may have wondered why I haven't mentioned weight loss very much as part of this plan. Here's where that comes in. It's take the pressure off time ...

## THE STRESS & WEIGHT CONNECTION

Linda Stone is a highly respected writer and trend consultant. She is mostly known for her pioneering work at Apple and Microsoft, in high technology. Since retiring from Microsoft, she has become better known for coining the phrase 'email apnea'.

She became aware that she routinely held her breath while checking her email so decided to people watch to see if others did the same. They do. She noticed it mainly among office workers, who frequently held their breath while working.

She checked with leading doctors to find out if breath holding and shallow breathing can affect a person's health - especially when done day in, day out. Apparently it really can.

One of the many doctors she consulted with was Dr Margaret Chesney, from the National Institute of Health (NIH). Dr Chesney had proved in her own research with another NIH scientist, Dr David Anderson, that breath holding and hyperventilating (fast breathing) alter the body's oxygen, carbon dioxide and nitrous oxide balance and contributes '*significantly*' to stress-related diseases. This is because anything other than good, deep, natural breathing can trigger the erroneously named 'fight or flight'[9] stress response. It's the body's natural reaction to perceived danger - and it thinks that you holding your breath (as you would do if you saw a large predator coming towards you at speed) is a sign that you have seen something potentially dangerous.

If your 'fight or flight' response is triggered, you will experience a number of changed body processes, involving the sympathetic nervous system and the adrenal-cortical system. Amongst other things, this causes the liver to put glucose and cholesterol in the bloodstream so you have the energy to run away from the danger, and adrenaline will flood your system, giving you strength. Your heart rate will increase, as will your blood pressure. This is your body speeding up, tensing up, and becoming more alert. You may feel a little cold - that's the veins in your skin constricting so the blood in them can be diverted to

---

[9] The fight or flight stress response is now sometimes called the fight, flight, or freeze stress response. www.stressstop.com/stress-tips/articles/fight-flight-or-freeze-response-to-stress.php

major muscle groups. You may notice the hairs on your arms stand upright - due to the muscles tensing up. In extreme cases, you might need to rush to the bathroom - making you lighter and more able to run. Non-essential systems will shut down - possibly causing indigestion and burping as the body doesn't consider digestion to be a high priority when facing an imminent attack.

If all this happens to you while you're working or simply checking your emails it's more than a little inconvenient. You don't want a racing heart, tense muscles (which get painful after a while), the urge to run away or run to the bathroom.

It's a classic stress response but it's a chicken-and-egg thing - which came first, the stress or the shallow breathing/breath holding?

If you have experienced any of the stress symptoms, or have found yourself reacting unusually badly to stressful situations of late, you may find that the breathing routine here will help. Focusing on this breathing routine will regulate your sympathetic nervous system. Do the routine twice daily for the 10 days of this plan, while doing your brushing routine.

## HOW TO BREATHE

Breathe in, breathe out. Repeat. It seems so simple so why do so many of us get it wrong? It's all to do with stress.

If you watch a baby breathe you'll see that the movement doesn't involve the chest, it's the abdomen. This 23 second video shows it perfectly:

**http://bit.ly/babybreathing**

That's how we should all breathe but life tends to get more stressful as we grow up and clothes become more constricting. We stop expanding our abdomens and move only our chests, or even just our upper chests and shoulders. This prevents us from taking in enough air to get adequate oxygen, and can cause a stress reaction.

If you're ever done martial arts, yoga, or taken a singing class, you may have been taught deep breathing and experienced the tremendous benefits. It really has the power to make you feel wonderful within just a couple of minutes. Sort of calm and serene and clean on the inside.

Linda Stone wonders if modern-day health problems could be related to our poor breathing habits. She says[10]:

> *"Now I want to know: Is it only the Big Mac that makes us fat? Or, are we more obese and diabetic because of a combination of holding our breath off and on all day and then failing to move when our bodies have prepared us to do so?*
>
> *Can fifteen minutes of diaphragmatic breathing before a meal tune us in to when we're full?...*
> *Can daily breathing exercises contribute to helping reduce asthma, ADD, depression, obesity, and a host of other stress-related conditions?"*

There's something very exciting yet natural about the possibility that deep breathing could make us feel better. It makes sense.

---

[10] www.huffingtonpost.com/linda-stone/just-breathe-building-the_b_85651.html

Breathing properly will help relax both your mind and your body and get proper oxygen supplies to your whole system. The breathing routine you are going to do with your skin brushing, done twice daily, will improve the strength of your diaphragm and the quality of your breathing. It will make you more likely to continue.

We're going to be doing diaphragmatic breathing - that is breathing that really gets the diaphragm moving. The diaphragm is a large dome of muscle and tendon that separates the chest cavity and the abdominal cavity. It is attached to the ribs and takes its shape from how it is attached and from the position of the organs below it (liver, stomach, colon, etc.).

You may have heard people talk about deep breathing before, this is what they mean, actively engaging the diaphragm. It will be moving anyway, we're just going to work it harder to take in more air. Moving the diaphragm downwards causes a vacuum in the lungs, which will pull more air in.

Frankly, it has never helped me at all when people have told me to 'belly breathe' or breathe deep into my abdomen. I have enough of a grasp of anatomy to know that my lungs aren't in my belly and it isn't possible to breathe air into my abdomen.

What is happening is that, when the diaphragm moves downwards and pulls more air into the lungs, the air spreads out throughout the lungs from the center, where it comes in through the bronchial tubes. I find that more helpful to think about than 'belly breathing'.

So when I breathe I think about my diaphragm moving towards, pulling my ribs out to the sides to allow all that nourishing air to flow into my lungs.

It was my daughter who eventually taught me how to breathe properly. She took years of singing lessons so it is completely natural for her to breathe using her diaphragm.

# DEEP BREATHING EXERCISE

I have read about deep breathing exercises many times over the years but none have 'clicked' in the way that this one did, that my daughter taught me. She studied at Stagecoach Theater School and was taught how to use her diaphragm properly and now does it without thinking - taking deep, natural breaths, like a baby does, without it being forced.

I caught her watching me one day when we were watching TV and asked why. She said she was monitoring my breathing and thought I was breathing too shallowly. She explained that using just the upper part of the lungs is quite common (especially for women with incorrectly-fitted bras apparently!) and can cause numerous health problems.

A good way to think about it is to breathe without worrying about whether you look fat! Lots of people have a habit of holding their abdomen in all the time, which makes them breathe shallowly. No-one has to tell a sleeping baby or puppy to expand their tummy when they breathe in, they just do it naturally because they aren't stressing about it.

I said that I had tried breathing exercises before but they only worked at the time, and afterwards I went back to my poor breathing habits.

She assured me that I wouldn't after her lesson! Here it is:

Your lungs sort of sit on your diaphragm, which is a thick band of muscle that lives at the bottom of your ribcage. Most breathing exercises get you to expand your ribcage or force air in or out of your lungs. That's counterproductive. Forget about your lungs, your chest, and your ribcage and focus instead on your diaphragm.

Take a slow, deep breath and think about your diaphragm expanding downwards and moving your ribs out to the sides. Let the breath go naturally, as it wants to, at the end of the inhale.

Most people teach deep breathing incorrectly by telling people to focus on expanding their abdomen. People start to feel that they are wrong if their chests move when they breathe - they're not! Your diaphragm is attached to your ribs so, when it moves, your ribs naturally move too, to the sides. So the whole of your torso should move when you are breathing, really, including your upper chest.

What shouldn't move are your shoulders. That's why we're going to start our breathing routine on the floor, so they are completely relaxed and not pushing to get in on the action!

People worry whether or not they're doing deep breathing correctly. That's adding stress about a perfectly natural process.

## THE BREATHING ROUTINE

Society on the whole has terrible posture. We slump over computers, slouch in armchairs, and drive hunched over our steering wheels. This all affects our breathing as our lungs don't have room and our abdomens can't expand properly.

If you look at people in the street, you won't see many who have their shoulders in the right place. Instead, their shoulders are rounded forward, causing the backs of their hands to show at the front of their bodies, instead of their arms hanging at their sides, with the sides of their hands and thumbs showing.

So starting your breathing routine sitting or standing up isn't going to be ideal, because the chances are that your shoulders will be rounded forward. So here's what to try:

Lie on your back on the floor with your calves resting on something like a coffee table. Your thighs should be vertical, with your knees pointing at the ceiling. Your calves should be horizontal on the coffee table, with your feet relaxed. In this position your shoulders sit in their proper place and your neck, back and abdominal muscles can relax. This will prevent you from using the neck and shoulders when you are breathing, and enable you to learn where you should be breathing from. Stay in this position for a minute or so, just relaxing and becoming aware of your breathing. Try to notice what it is doing without influencing it - not easy!

Put your left hand on your abdomen just over and above your belly button. Take a few slightly longer and deeper breaths than you are used to. Inhale through your nose and exhale through your mouth. The chances are that your hand won't move very much and you may be aware that your chest does. That's fine, for now. As the diaphragm is largely muscle, it gets stronger and more capable the more you exercise it - and it gets weak and floppy when you don't - so we're going to exercise it. Eventually, diaphragmatic breathing will become second-nature to you.

Inhale and think about your diaphragm (which is beneath your hand) expanding downwards. Focus on drawing your breath in low into the base of your lungs, where your diaphragm is making room for their expansion by easing your ribs out to the sides. Do this over a slow count of 4.

Hold it for just a couple of seconds but don't close your throat, stay relaxed, and then...

Exhale (slowly, through your mouth) and think about your diaphragm beginning to rise again as your lungs release air and your ribs relax back into place. Exhale over a slow count of 4. You can slightly draw in your abdomen if it helps.

Importantly, don't take another deep breath, just relax and allow your breathing to go back to normal. Most deep breathing exercises don't do this, they get you to do lots of deep breaths together, which can be a bit overwhelming for a body that isn't used to all that oxygen.

After half a minute or so, take another deep breath.

The more you do this, the more likely it is that you hand will start to move as you breathe in, indicating that you are breathing using your diaphragm, not your chest and shoulders.

When your diaphragm moves down with the in-breath, the organs underneath it need to move, so your abdomen expands. This allows you to get a really full breath of air and thoroughly oxygenate yourself.

It is why people who habitually only breathe from their upper chests - i.e. people whose chests and shoulders move when they breathe - are more likely to suffer from the problems I spoke about earlier which are associated with stress. They simply aren't getting enough oxygen and their bodies think there's danger just around the corner.

## INCORPORATE DEEP BREATHING INTO YOUR SKIN BRUSHING ROUTINE

Do some deep breathing before you start your brushing routine, each time. Take the time to take two deep breaths, at least.

Once you are used to engaging your diaphragm, you can progress to doing some deep breathing while sitting or standing. Again, go slowly, you don't want to topple over.

Eventually, you'll be able to carry on with the deep breathing while you're doing your brushing – whatever position you have to twist yourself into!

If you combine your brushing with your breathing, it can have a very calming effect on the nervous system. Two or three brush strokes per inhale is better than trying to do one brush stroke each inhale.

## BREATHING WHILE EXERCISING

Breathing teachers say we should breathe in when moving away from the pull of gravity and breathe out when moving towards the pull of gravity.

This is a good thing to remember - especially in the gym when you can't think if you should be breathing in or out when pushing the weight away from you (in!).

# FAQ ABOUT DEEP BREATHING

## *Is it normal to feel dizzy when doing deep breathing?*

Yes, absolutely. It can be because your body isn't used to taking in so much oxygen. It can also be because you are breathing out too slowly and aren't getting oxygen in quickly enough, so try shortening the length of your exhale.

When you feel dizzy, have a little break from deep breathing for a few seconds while your body acclimatizes. The dizziness periods will get shorter and less frequent and eventually disappear.

For this reason, though, it isn't a great idea to practice deep breathing while doing something important such as driving.

## *How often should I practice?*

If you can, practice twice daily before and during your skin brushing sessions.

Throughout the day, whenever you remember, just think about slowing down your inhales now and again, sitting up, and rolling your shoulders back into position. This will allow you to breathe more deeply when you are working and not even thinking about deep breathing.

# CHAPTER 11
## STEP THREE – START SKIN BRUSHING

☾☽

NOW FOR THE fun part! If you haven't got your brush yet don't panic, you can start doing the movements with your hands.

You're going to be doing this every morning (hopefully) for the next ten days. Then afterwards you can carry on with daily brushing or just do it a couple of times a week. Whatever fits in best with your routine.

You can increase to twice a day if you wish but I wouldn't start with that or you could get a cleansing reaction. Stick to once per day for the first ten days and see how you feel before increasing the frequency of brushing.

For the first few days, stick to brushing each section of the body just twice (once near the nearest cluster of lymph glands, then again covering the same area but from slightly further away).

After a couple of days, if you aren't experiencing any side-effects, you can increase this to four strokes on each section.

If you have a brand new brush it may be a little stiff so be extra careful until it has softened a little. Giving it a wash in warm water (and dry near but not on a heat source) will help.

# THE [NEW] BRUSHING ROUTINE

As I mentioned earlier, most people advise starting at the feet when skin brushing. Forget that! We are going to draw on the wisdom of lymphatic drainage experts, who generally start at the upper chest for a whole body treatment. That enables us to stimulate the big lymphatic ducts first and make way for the increased lymph flow that we are going to cause.

If you've done skin brushing in the past there's no need to be concerned that you've been wasting your time - you haven't. I'm sure you enjoyed many of the wonderful benefits that skin brushing brings such as smoother & firmer skin, improved cellulite, and more energy. You just won't have been stimulating your lymphatic system as effectively as you will be doing with my new method.

If you haven't done skin brushing before, I suggest you use the brush only on your hands and feet for the first few days. Use your hands for the rest of your body. This is for three reasons:

1. Many of the areas that are rich in lymphatic glands are actually quite tender - the neck, upper chest, armpits, groin. Learning to massage over these areas is better than jumping straight in with a brush, as you will be more aware of the pressure you need to apply.

2. Hand and foot skin is tougher and less likely to react badly to the feel of the brush. It will enable you to get used to

wielding the brush and the amount of pressure that your skin will tolerate.

3. It will get your body used to the feeling of the skin brushing movements but using the hands, so it won't be as stimulating as it will be in a few days' time, when we'll start using the brush. So you can start to stimulate your lymph but in a gentle way that shouldn't bring on a Heixheimer/cleansing reaction - if you are adequately hydrated.

So have a go using your hands first, using light movements - not pressure. If you used a normal massaging movement you would be pressing down on the initial lymph vessels. We want to use a very light stretching movement so we open those vessels up, not squish them. That's why dry skin brushing is better than other methods of self-massage. Better than a loofah, which can irritate the skin; better than one of those little plastic poufs, which don't move the skin; better than a traditional bath brush, which is too soft to have much effect on the circulation.

## THE FULL BODY ROUTINE

Think of your body as being split with invisible lines down the middle, across the collarbone area, and across the waist. These lines mark where we will be brushing on, from, and to.

Generally:

- ➤ Brush in the direction of center to outside of the body;
- ➤ Brush towards the nearest cluster of lymph glands;
- ➤ Start nearest the cluster, brushing towards it, and then pick the brush up and move it further away, then brush towards the cluster, covering the same area as the first stroke. This is the piping bag effect.

**COLLARBONE:**

Start just below the neck, on the collarbone. Brush in three small circles from the center of the collarbone out towards the left shoulder. Then three small circles from the center out towards the right shoulder.

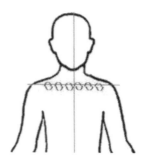

**NECK:**

You're going to be brushing the front of your neck in three sections, starting from the center and brushing once from halfway between your chin and throat, then once from your chin to your throat first, then moving out and brushing from the midpoint of the left lower jaw to the clavicle in two strokes (the first from the halfway point, the second the full section), then from just below the ear to where the neck joins the shoulder in two strokes (again, from halfway and the full section).

Repeat on the right side of your neck.

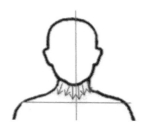

**FACE:**

Brush your face very gently, or use your hands if your facial skin is too sensitive. Brush once from nose to chin, just to the left of your nose, then – covering the same path – from forehead to chin. Move the brush out halfway towards your left ear and brush once downwards from cheek to the centre of your left lower jaw. Then once from the midpoint on the left of your forehead down to your lower jaw. Then brush from just in front of your left ear down to the outer edge of your jaw and then from your left temple down to the outer edge of your jaw.

Finally, brush outwards from the center of the left side of your face out towards the ear, once from the forehead, once from the nose, and once from the chin.

Repeat the downward and outward movements on the right side of your face.

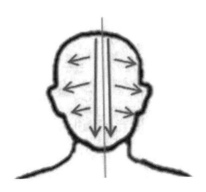

**BACK OF NECK AND UPPER BACK:**

For most people, it is too difficult to try to do the half section/full section brushing on the back of the neck. Just brush twice from hairline to the top of your back.

At the back of the neck, brush twice from the center of the base of your hairline on the left-hand side, downwards and slightly out towards your left shoulder, stopping at the top of your back. Then move the brush back to your hairline towards your left ear and brush once down towards your shoulder. Add a third section, more towards your ear, if you have a large neck (or a small brush).

Finally, sweep the brush across the top of your back, from just below your neck right across your shoulder, twice.

Repeat on your right side.

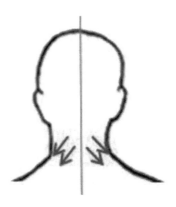

**ARMS:**

We're going to split the upper and then lower arms into four sections – inner, upper, outer, and under.

**Upper Arm:**

Lift your left arm up and brush the inner part once from ½-way between your inner elbow and your armpit, then once all the way from your elbow to your armpit. Brush once on the upper part of your arm from half way between the outer fold of your elbow and your shoulder, then all the way from your elbow bone to your shoulder. Then brush the outer part of your arm (the 'bingo wing') from ½-way up the arm to the top where it meets the body, then from the elbow bone up over the same area. Finally, brush the under part of your arm from half way up to your armpit, then the full length of the upper arm to your armpit.

**Lower Arm:**

Brush the inner part of your arm along the bone from wrist (below the base of your thumb) to inner elbow, then from tip of index finger, over your thumb and up the length of your lower arm to your inner elbow. Then brush from the top of your wrist up to your elbow, and from the tip of your middle finger over the back of your hand and up to your elbow; Move to the outer bone and brush from your wrist (just below the base of your pinkie) up to your elbow, and from the tip of your pinkie up to your elbow. Finally, brush the under part of your lower arm from inner wrist to elbow, then from the tips of your fingers, over your palm and up to your inner elbow.

Repeat on your right arm.

[Optional] Brush your entire arm, again in 4 long, sweeping sections, from the tips of the fingers to the armpit or shoulder.

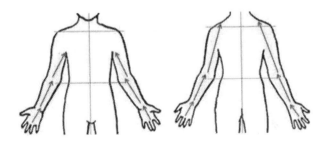

**UPPER CHEST**:

From the center of the chest, just below the left clavicle, brush once straight downwards. Lift the brush and place it just below your clavicle an inch or two towards your left shoulder. Brush once downwards and towards your left armpit. Lift the brush and place it just below the outer part of your clavicle. Brush once downwards directly towards your left armpit.

Repeat on the right side of your chest.

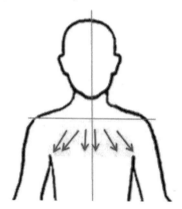

**BREASTS**:

If your breasts aren't too sensitive, brush from just to the left of the center of the body out towards the left armpit, twice.

Repeat on the right side.

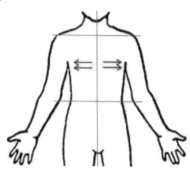

## TORSO:

We're splitting each half of the upper torso into three sections. Put the brush just above and slightly left of your bellybutton and brush upwards towards your breasts twice, stopping just below the curve of left breast (this is for men too – men have breasts!). Move the brush half-way between your bellybutton and side (on your waistline) and brush upwards twice to underneath your left breast. Now put the brush out almost to your side (still on your waistline) and brush twice upwards right up to your armpit.

Repeat on your right front torso.

Now repeat on your left back, brushing upwards and slightly outwards (because of the angle), again brush twice on each of the three sections, starting at the centre, then towards the side, then almost on the side again.

Repeat on your right back.

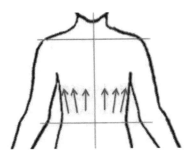

## ABDOMEN:

Starting just above the bellybutton, brush in a small circle in an anticlockwise direction around your bellybutton (i.e. towards your left side). Keep brushing for two more circles, each one bigger than the last. The last one should cover the whole of your abdomen.

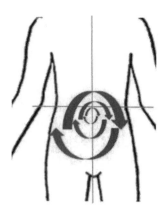

## HIPS & GLUTES:

We're going to brush over the butt outwards towards the hip in three sections.

Brush outwards from the center of your body over the butt, ending at the hip, in three sections from the waistline down. Brush each section twice.

Repeat on the right side.

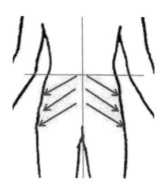

## LEGS:

We'll handle the legs in two parts – thighs first then calves/feet. Like the arms, we're going to split them into four sections.

### Thighs:

Starting at the inside of the left thigh, brush upwards towards the groin twice, once from halfway between the inside of the knee and the groin and once all the way from the inner knee to the groin. Then move to the top of the thigh. Brush upwards and slightly inwards towards the groin twice, once from halfway between the knee and the groin and once from the knee to the groin. Then start at the outside of the thigh. Brush twice up towards the hip, once from halfway between the outer knee and the hip and once all the way up from knee to hip. Finally, do the back of the thigh. Brush twice upwards towards the butt, once from halfway between the back of the knee and the butt and once all the way up from the back of the knee.

### Calves & feet:

These are easiest to do sitting down. Starting on the inside edge of the left calf, brush twice upwards towards from halfway between the inside of the foot and the inner knee, then all the way from the inner foot to the inner knee.. Then move to the top of the foot and calf. Brush twice up towards the knee, first from halfway between the toes and the knee, then all the way up from the tips of the toes to the knee. Move to the outside of the calf and brush twice from the outer foot up towards the outer knee, first from halfway between the tip of the little toe and the outside of the knee, then all the way up from the little toe to the knee. Move to the underneath of the calf. Brush twice, once from halfway between the heel of your foot and the back of the knee, then once all the way from the heel to the knee. Finally, prop your foot up and brush the sole (if you aren't too ticklish!) from toes to heel, three times.

Finish your left leg by brushing once all the way up the inside edge of the leg, from foot to groin; once from the toes and top of the foot up to the groin; once from the outside edge of your foot up to your hip; and once from the toes on the underneath of your foot, over the sole and up the back of your leg, ending at the groin.

Repeat on the right leg.

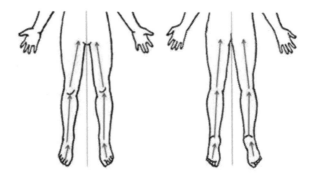

That's the full all-over body skin brushing routine. Reading it makes it seem much more complicated that it actually is. You'll soon get used to it and be able to do it without referring to these instructions.

If there are parts of your body that you can't reach, don't worry about them and just move to parts that you can reach. You may find that you become more flexible with this routine and are able to reach a little further but, if not, don't worry. You're still stimulating your whole body when brushing other areas.

The full routine, done quite vigorously, can be a bit like an aerobic workout. Indeed you can treat it as such, once you're used to it. It should zip up your energy for the day, done in the morning.

But what about people who don't have the time or freedom to brush in the mornings? Read on...

# CHAPTER 12
# THE SUPER RELAXING
# BEFORE BED BRUSHING ROUTINE

ෆ৪৪১

PERHAPS YOUR MORNINGS are a frantic whirl of bagging lunches and shoving children out of the door towards the bus, before tumbling into your car and stabbing some makeup on while you drive to work.

Maybe you have other commitments or demanding family members and the chance of getting any time alone in the morning is as likely as winning the lottery. So you might give a hollow laugh at the prospect of trying to cram anything else into your routine.

Yet the magazines and websites that shout about how wonderful skin brushing is always say that it should be done in the morning before showering.

Well I've some good news for you. It is possible to do a skin brushing routine that you not only don't have to do in the morning, but that can help you relax and get a better night's sleep.

Some of my friends have young children and the only time they manage to carve for themselves is in the quiet time after the children have gone to bed. By then they're generally too exhausted to do anything other than slouch in front of the TV in a daze.

I devised the super relaxing before bed brushing routine to help them and everyone else who can only find some time for themselves in the time before going to bed.

Vigorous brushing will, of course, stimulate the blood circulation and give you an energetic buzz. So the before bed routine is designed to be slow and soothing. It will work on the nervous system to help prepare you for bed. Done regularly as part of your winding down routine before going to bed, it will even help you sleep.

First of all, you need to prepare by buying a bottle of one of the sedative/relaxing essential oils.

---

### SEDATIVE/RELAXING ESSENTIAL OILS

Benzoin, Chamomile, Lavender,
Marjoram[Sweet], Neroli, Orange,
Vetiver, Ylang-Ylang.

---

You don't need more than one oil, any of the ones in the box above is very effective on its own. If you happen to have a few bottles already, then you can use a combination by adding a few drops of each to a clean bottle and using one drop of this blend in your bowl of warm water.

The cheapest oils tend to be orange and lavender. Chamomile is quite expensive. Marjoram is my favorite.

Here's what to do:

1. Put some warm water in a small bowl and take it to your bedroom, together with a bottle of a calming essential oil. When you get there ...

2. Begin by dimming the lights, if you can. If you have a bedside lamp, you could switch that on and turn off the overhead light.

3. Undress and sit down in a comfortable chair or on your bed.

4. Put a drop of the oil in the bowl of warm water. Hold it under your chin, so you can smell the oil but so it isn't too close to your nose (which could damage your sensitive nasal passages), then ...

5. Take two wonderful, relaxing deep breaths, expanding your chest out to the sides as you breathe in and feeling everything relax and soften as you breathe out. Understand that oils that are taken in via the nose reach the brain quicker than via any other method. That means that the properties of the oil are already working.

6. Put the bowl down (in a safe place!), take your brush and start, as usual, at your collarbones. Using light pressure, brush using slow circles out towards the left shoulder, then out towards the right.

7. Carry on with the routine, using light, slow, and soothing strokes. Keep breathing deeply as you brush (if you remember!). Try to coordinate the brush strokes with your breath: Three or four strokes per in-breath or out-breath

(or whatever is comfortable for you).

8. Use very light, circular strokes on your abdomen. You don't want to stimulate your bowl overnight!

9. When you get to the legs, be careful not to brush the soles of the feet too virogously. There are over 7,000 nerve endings in the feet and, because they tend to be quite tough, I've noticed that a lot of people brush them quite firmly, which can be over-stimulating at night.

10. Finish your session by putting your brush down and picking up your bowl again and doing a few more deep breaths. Rinse the bowl out afterwards so no-one (human or animal) is tempted to drink from it.

---

**OPTIONAL EXTRA**

If you have a suitable carrier oil - that's a regular vegetable oil, not an essential oil - you could put some in a small bottle (around 10ml size) and add 2 or 3 drops of your calming essential oil(s).

This is great for massaging into your temples, neck and shoulders before bed, to further help you relax and drift off to sleep naturally.

**SUITABLE CARRIER OILS:**

*Grapeseed, almond, coconut, jojoba, apricot.*

This routine will be enough to gently encourage and support your body's natural detoxification processes, exfoliate and tone your skin, and give your muscles some extra freshly oxygenated blood. If you keep your mind calm and your breathing slow and deep you will stay relaxed and be nicely warm and ready for sleep.

# CHAPTER 13
## THE SUPER FAST, 'LATE FOR WORK' BRUSHING ROUTINE

 C380

KATE WAS ONE of the beta testers for this skin brushing plan and experienced fantastic benefits from it - firmer skin, more energy, a healthy glow. When she next came to me for a massage it was because she was feeling depressed and run down and thought the massage would pick her up. She had moved house to in order to be nearer a good school for her son, but now had a longer commute to work and hadn't done any skin brushing for weeks. Listening to the extraordinary list of things she had to do in the mornings, I could understand why!

So I came up with the super fast brushing routine to see if she could manage to fit that into her busy day a couple of times a week. She did and is delighted to be brushing regularly again, because she has made it a habit.

Now here it is for you. This works because you have already got the benefit of using the full routine and know how and where on your body to brush. You don't need to brush every inch of your body numerous times to get the benefit of skin brushing. This quick routine will get your circulation zipped up and leave you tingling and raring to go.

Use light but quick brushing strokes. We're going to cover each section with just one full stroke, not split halfway.

**CLAVICLE:**

Brush across the top of the left clavicle from center to shoulder in three small circles. Repeat on the right. 6 seconds.

This is a really important area because of where the lymph drains back into the venus system so we're doing the full number of brush strokes here.

**NECK:**

Brush in three downward strokes, starting from just left of the center of the next and brushing once from chin to throat first, then moving out and brushing from the midpoint of the left lower jaw to the clavicle once, then from just below the ear to where the neck joins the shoulder once. Repeat on the right side of your neck. 6 seconds.

**FACE:**

Gently brush your face (or use your hands if your facial skin is too sensitive). Brush once from forehead to chin, then once from halfway along the hairline down to the center of the lower jaw, and from just above the outer edge of the eyebrow down to the outer edge of the jaw. Finally, brush from the center of the face out towards the ear, once from the forehead, once from the nose, and once from the chin. Repeat on the right side of your face. 10 seconds.

**BACK OF NECK**:

At the back of the neck, brush once from the center of the base of your hairline straight down to the top of your back, then move the brush back to your hairline towards your left ear and brush once down towards your shoulder, then at the other side towards your right ear brush down once from the hairline down towards your shoulder. 3 seconds.

**UPPER CHEST**:

From the center of the chest, just below the clavicle, brush once downwards towards the area between your breasts and twice from the center out towards your armpit. Repeat on the right side of your chest. 6 seconds.

**LEFT UPPER ARM**:

Lift your left arm and brush once from your inner elbow to your armpit (covering the inner soft part of your arm), then once on the top of your arm from the area between the inner and outer elbow, then once from your elbow bone, brushing up towards your shoulder and beyond, finishing at the back of your shoulder. So you will have covered the upper arm in three brush strokes. 3 seconds.

**LEFT LOWER ARM & HAND**:

With your palm facing down, brush once from your fingertips over the top of your hand up to the crook of your elbow, then turn your palm up and brush from the fingertips up to your inner elbow. 2 seconds.

[Optional] Brush your entire arm, again in 3 sections, from the tips of the fingers to the armpit or shoulder. 3 seconds.

**RIGHT ARM**:

Repeat on your upper and lower right arm. 5 seconds.

**TORSO**:

Put the brush on your bellybutton and brush upwards once, stopping between your breasts. Move the brush half-way between your bellybutton and side (on your waistline) and brush upwards once to underneath your left breast. Now put the brush on your side (still on your waistline) and brush once upwards right up to your armpit. Repeat on the back, brushing upwards and slightly outwards (because of the angle), again three times, starting at the centre, then towards the side, then on the side again. 6 seconds.

Repeat on your right torso, front and back. 6 seconds.

**ABDOMEN**:

Starting just above the bellybutton, brush in a small circle in an anticlockwise direction around your bellybutton (i.e. towards your left side). Keep brushing for two more circles, each one bigger than the last. The last one should cover the whole of your abdomen. 3 seconds.

**HIPS & GLUTES**:

Brush once from the center of the back, just below the waistline, out and slightly down towards the hip. Then move the brush down the spine and brush from just above the top of the butt, out towards the left hip. Then across the butt. 3 seconds.

Repeat, brushing three times towards the right hip.

**LEFT THIGH**:

Starting at the inside of the left knee, brush once upwards towards the groin once. Then start on the knee and brush upwards and slightly inwards towards the groin. Then start at the outside of the knee and brush once up towards the hip.

Finally, start from the back of the knee and brush once upwards towards the butt. 4 seconds.

**LEFT CALF:**

Starting on the inside edge of the foot (the arch), brush once upwards towards the inner knee. Then move to the top of the foot and brush once up from the toes to the knee. Move to the outside of the leg and brush once up from the outer foot up towards the knee. Finally, pick up your foot and brush from the toes, over the sole, and up the back of the calf, stopping at the back of the knee. 4 seconds.

Finish your left leg - if you have time - by brushing once all the way up the inside edge of the leg, from foot to groin; once from the toes and top of the foot up to the groin; once from the outside edge of your foot up to your hip; and once up the back of your leg (you can incorporate the sole if you wish but I prefer to do this standing and start from my heel).

**RIGHT LEG:**

Repeat on the right leg. 12 seconds.

Total time: Under one and a half minutes. It's probably the best one and a half minutes you can invest in yourself and it is so easy. It makes you feel energized and ready to hit the day running.

For an extra boost, put a drop of an energizing essential oil into a basin of warm water and do your skin brushing routine in the bathroom. Breathe in the fragrant vapors before, during, and after your brushing.

Then you could drip a washcloth into the water, swish it around, and wring it out, Rub it all over your body (well, all the bits you can reach!) to get extra benefits from the oil.

The citrus oils are all energizing and most have the advantage of being inexpensive. Orange and Lemon are generally the cheapest. Use them on their own or blended with others. I use orange, lemon, & bergamot together.

---

### ENERGIZING ESSENTIAL OILS

*Bergamot, Eucalyptus, Grapefruit, Ginger, Lemon, Lime, Orange, Rosemary.*

# CHAPTER 14
# WHAT NOT TO DO

ೞ

Y OU'VE ALREADY READ about my bad experiences of doing too much too quickly. I don't like to focus on negatives but let's look at the things you shouldn't do to make certain that this skin brushing plan is going to work for you.

## 1. STOP 'SHOULD-ING' ON YOURSELF!

We all do it. We tell ourselves we 'should' do this, 'should not' have done that. We put burdens on our minds and bodies all the time. This is a detox, yes, but it is more of a plan of abundance than a plan of deprivation.

This plan is going to really benefit your body but it won't have the full effect if your mind isn't on board. Getting out of the 'should' - or 'I must' - mentality is the first step in letting go of old, limiting, stressy thought patterns.

Fit your skin brushing in around your regular lifestyle. This isn't another thing you have to try to squeeze onto your mountainous

'To Do' list, it isn't yet another chore that you may or may not get around to. See it as a fun, exhilarating new habit that you're taking up that's going to make you feel great, give you glowing skin, and have people questioning what you're doing/eating/not eating that's giving you such energy and charisma.

## 2. DON'T FEEL LIKE YOU'RE ON A TRADITIONAL DETOX

This plan is about supporting your body's natural detoxification systems - especially the lymphatic system. Detoxing and dieting promote feelings of deprivation, which result in stress - and, generally, overeating or at least indulging in unhelpful foods and drinks.

If you suspect that this is a problem for you, I highly recommend the book *The Cortisol Connection* by Shawn Talbott. It clearly demonstrates how stress causes us not only to gain weight but also prevents us from losing weight. Cortisol is a hormone that the body produces when under stress. Like its more famous cousin, adrenaline, it appears when there's an emergency, or a dangerous situation.

We may not think we lead a dangerous life but our bodies do. Poor lighting, excess noise, being unable to rest when we need to, not being able to punch someone on the nose who has cut us up in traffic - these are all high-level stressors.

Cortisol starts circulating to enable the body to deal with the danger, or run away from it. That means diverting precious energy away from non-essential things.

According to Shawn Talbott:

> *"Cortisol acts as a potent signal to the brain to increase appetite and cravings for certain foods, especially carbohydrates and fats (because of their high calorie levels).*
>
> *Cortisol also acts as a signal to our fat cells to hold on to as much fat as they can and to release as little fat as possible, even in the face of our attempts to reduce calorie intake for weight loss.*
>
> *It also alters the body's metabolic rate by blocking the effects of many of our most important metabolic hormones, including insulin (so blood-sugar levels suffer and carb cravings follow); serotonin (so we feel fatigued and depressed); growth hormones testosterone and estrogen (so our sex drive falls and we rarely feel 'in the mood')."*

If you read through that quotation again you will see that increased cortisol means increased appetite, increased cravings, fat retention, reduced metabolic rate (which means weight gain, bloating, muscle loss), blood sugar crashes, depression, sleepiness, and bone-wearying body aches. This is serious stuff.

Cortisol is convinced it is serious stuff too - and that we're about to need all our body's reserves of fat in order to have the reserves for the battle that is obviously upcoming or we wouldn't be so stressed.

It thinks we're constantly about to take part in a battle if we:

- ➤ Don't get enough sleep.
- ➤ Over or under eat.
- ➤ Spend more time under artificial lights than natural daylight.
- ➤ Hold our tongue and choke down our emotions rather than dealing with situations.
- ➤ Use stimulants to keep us going instead of resting - stimulants include caffeine, sugar, artificial sweeteners, drugs, loud music, bright lights, TV, computers, and more.
- ➤ Don't deal with conflict.
- ➤ Aren't assertive.

That means cortisol is telling the body there's an emergency situation about to take place and not to release any fat from where it's stored in the fat cells. The inability to lose weight when you are desperately trying to is in itself a stressor, sending cortisol into overdrive and the fat cells to go into lockdown.

Even if you aren't trying to lose weight, cortisol is bad news as it puts your body on permanent alert, causing fatigue, muscle pain, nervous tension, insomnia, and more.

Stress is what causes cortisol to rise and many experts say that good stress is as bad as bad stress. However that isn't strictly true. It is more our **reaction** to stress than the stress itself. We can train ourselves to not over-react to stress.

There's a wonderful TED talk by Kelly McGonigal about how to make stress your friend:

**www.ted.com/talks/kelly_mcgonigal_how_to_ma ke_stress_your_friend.html**

She found that stress is bad for people who believe it is doing them harm. They have an average 43% increased risk of dying after a particularly stressful event. People who experience a lot of stress but don't believe it is harming them have ***no*** increased risk of dying. Wow. It is what we believe it is.

The Oxford English Dictionary defines stress as:

> *A state of mental or emotional strain or tension resulting from adverse or demanding circumstances.*[11]

We recognize stress from adverse situations, such as a car wreck or the collapse of the financial markets, and often we realize we can do little about them so accept them fairly readily. Coping afterwards is the difficult part!

We don't always recognize stress from pleasant situations though, such as weddings, moving home, or changing job. These are still stressors and still cause a flood of cortisol.

The top stressors in life are often listed in the media. The Australian website SourceCentre[12] lists them as:

1.  Death of a loved one.
2.  Divorce/breakup.
3.  Losing a job - or being unable to find one.
4.  Financial worries/debts.
5.  Work stress.

---

11 Oxford English Dictionary
12 www.sourcecentre.net.au

6. Health issues.
7. Personal relationship issues.
8. Not having enough time.
9. Major life changes, such as moving home.
10. Conflict.

I think that numbers 6-10 are the ones most of us don't recognize and we carry on regardless, getting more and more stressed, snappy, forgetful, sick, and tired.

There are few things that I think are missing from that list but that should be fairly high up.

> **Extreme Dieting/Detoxing.** Trying to switch to a healthy lifestyle in such a bull-headed way that it puts our bodies on high stress alert. Your body, your mind, and your spirit have enough to deal with without you adding deprivation, cravings, punishing new habits, and food group or calorie restriction to their workload.

> Lack of **assertiveness**. Assertiveness isn't aggression. It isn't the modern "Because I'm worth it" attitude that shouts down others' needs in favor of our own. Assertiveness is recognizing that your needs are equal to the needs of others. It is the airplane oxygen mask lesson - you have to put on your own mask if you want to be capable of helping the person next to you. You have to meet your own needs first if you are going to be in any state to meet the needs of your loved ones, your professors, or your employer.

CS&O

Let's stop putting our bodies under excess stress. Let's forget all about diets and detoxes and concentrate on abundance and nourishment. Please take the next 10 days out from the regular rat race and choose to spend a few minutes each day nourishing your body and calming your mind through skin brushing and deep breathing.

Don't worry or even think about avoiding anything or cutting anything out of your diet. Once you have done the 10-day plan, you'll be in a better position to think about putting good stuff in to your diet and taking up new, gentle, healthier habits that will - hopefully - gradually edge out any unhealthy habits you have.

This is a body-friendly plan that will also benefit your mind and, without even trying, your spirit.

# CHAPTER 15
## EIGHT OTHER LIFESTYLE CHANGES TO ENJOY

CR෴

THERE ARE LOTS of health boosting naturopathic techniques that you can use at home. I've listed the ones here that I know and trust. These are good things that you can enjoy testing out, not more stressors to add to your 'To Do' list!

Do be careful of trying new techniques - remember my 'all or nothing' experiences of total overload. One thing at a time is less of a shock for the body. Ideally, try something new for 10 days to give yourself time to get used to it and before adding anything else new. Then you'll be sure that if you do have some sort of reaction, that it was that one thing. You won't have to turn detective to unravel which of the things you took up could have caused the problem!

Don't remove things from your diet or lifestyle with an 'all or nothing' approach either. If you want to give something up – say caffeine – then do it gently after you have nourished your body with its new skin brushing routine. Then you can start cutting down, mixing half and half decaf with regular, etc.

If you love a new technique, schedule it on your calendar so that you make regular appointments with yourself to do it. If you have to cancel an appointment it's no biggie, just reschedule.

You could refer back to this chapter when you need a boost from time to time, or use some of the suggestions as treats for yourself when you would normally buy something such as chocolate or alcohol!

# 1. GET GOOD QUALITY SLEEP

Getting enough sleep is the first step towards a healthier life - it improves your mind, body, and spirit. Sadly, many of us not only ignore our body's cries for sleep, we actually medicate against them. We eat sugar, caffeine, alcohol, and other stimulants, then wonder why we have trouble sleeping when it comes to bedtime.

It is natural for creatures to sleep more in the darker months of the year and be more active and alert during the lighter months. Modern lifestyles don't allow for that, though. We do the same things year-round with no allowance for the different needs we may have at different times of the year.

Many people complain of either needing too much sleep and waking unrefreshed or not being able to sleep.

Looking at it simply, we should try to go to bed earlier during the darker months of the year. Light stimulates our brains and hormones, it is effective at waking us and keeping us awake.

I have struggled with insomnia for years. Sometimes it is caused by pain, sometimes by tinnitus (ringing in the ears), sometimes by outside things that I can't control, often it is worries and unclassified concerns.

My solution was simple - an iPod! In the past, I would flick on the TV if I was awake a lot during the night. You can feel quite lonely, the only one awake in the long dark hours, and the company of the TV is welcome. That's the worst thing I could have done, though, as the light from a TV (like a computer) is the blue light that is very stimulating. Now I put on my iPod, which I am very familiar with and can use with my eyes closed. I load it with comedy shows (my favorite is *The Big Bang Theory*) that I have previously watched. That's important - if they are new episodes I want to open my eyes to see what's going on!

The combination of something familiar and funny relaxes me and allows me to listen without opening my eyes and allowing light in. This stops my brain from dwelling on problems, stops light entering and stimulating more wakefulness, and I drift off quickly. Very quickly, usually within a minute or two.

Sometimes, though, my wakefulness is longer and I can listen to a few episodes. That's fine. My body is getting rest even if my brain doesn't need sleep.

## Other tips to trick insomnia:

**Limit caffeine** - Everyone knows they shouldn't drink caffeine before bed but the time differs for everyone. Some people can only take caffeine in the morning, any later in the day will affect their sleep. If you have regular tussles with insomnia (and it can be bad enough to seem like a living nightmare, horrendous nights and zombie-like days), it may be worth reducing down until you just have a morning coffee. You would need to taper down gradually to avoid the crippling headaches that can accompany caffeine reduction.

**Get cold** - This works for some people. Throw off the bed covers and wait until you are cold before pulling them back and getting cozy. I drift off pretty quickly using this technique most of the time.

**Wet socks** - This sounds very odd but was taught to me by a herbalist that I worked with and it is surprisingly effective. Soak some socks in cold water, wring them out well, then put them on. Put a second, bigger, pair on top of them, then go to bed. This is similar to a technique naturopaths use to control fevers, where they will wrap a patient in a wet sheet.

**Avoid light before bed** - You may be more sensitive to light than other people. Stop watching TV or using computers, smartphones/tablets, etc., a few hours before bed. Turn the lights down and listen to music or read quietly. Take a warm (not hot, which can be stimulating) bath and have muted lights in the bathroom (candles are a good choice, they don't stimulate wakefulness, and it's the one place in the house where I don't worry about causing a fire with them!).

When you go to bed, don't switch on a bright overhead light, use a lamp if possible. Don't use bright lights if you have to go to the bathroom during the night either. Keep a torch by your bed. Obviously if you are prone to falls you may have to find other ways round this as lack of light would contribute to your likelihood of tripping.

I found out that my nighttime bathroom visit was a major contributor to my inability to get back to sleep. So now I make sure that the path from my bedroom to the bathroom is always kept clear and I can manage to get there without switching on a light or using a torch. If you do need a light on (safety is more important than a bit of light!), you could try shielding your eyes and/or using slightly dimmer bulbs in the lights you need to be on.

A drop of **essential oil** on your pillow can be helpful. Many people suggest lavender - which is excellent - but not everyone likes the smell. If you don't like the smell it certainly won't help you sleep! Try instead, the more powerful but lesser known marjoram. I keep a bottle of marjoram (also known as sweet marjoram, not the same thing as oregano) by my bed. It has a very calming effect on the nervous system and is particularly good for those nights when you go to bed with your stomach in a knot over some problem or stressor.

If you have a willing or bribable partner, a massage before bed can almost knock you out. Self-massage can also be effective:

> ➤ Take a teaspoon of vegetable oil such as grapeseed or almond and add one or two drops of the oil of your choice. You could put the oil blend in a container such as an egg-cup to make it easier and less likely to spill.

> ➤ Now put your nose over the egg-cup and take a breath.

> ➤ Then dip your fingers in the oil and place them on your neck at the outer edge of your jaw, crossed-over so your right hand is on the left side of your neck and your left hand on the right. There are lymph glands under there. Smooth your hands down your neck to the top of your chest, then lift off and put your fingers back up to the top of your neck but further along your jawbone towards your chin before smoothing down again. The idea is that you are smoothing the oils into your skin and massaging your lymph glands in the direction of the flow of lymph.

> ➤ Smooth your hands across your upper chest, working from the center outwards.

➢ If there is any oil left, dot a little under your nostrils and smooth some over your nose from the bridge, out to the cheeks.

➢ Any extra oil can be massaged into your hands and nails to give them a treat.

## Herbal Teas

Herbal teas aren't everyone's cup of tea! They can take some getting used to but it is worth persevering with them. The most inoffensive one is peppermint because it is a taste that many people are familiar with and can move onto without too much trauma.

Peppermint tea after a meal is good habit to start. The taste of peppermint makes you less likely to want something sweet, which can cause wakefulness if you eat late at night.

A word of warning with peppermint though. There are people who simply switch from having 6 or so cups of ordinary tea a day to having 6 cups of strong peppermint tea. Not a great idea. Peppermint relaxes smooth muscle and there are some smooth muscles you don't want to relax - mainly the one (actually a sphincter) that prevents the bowel from unloading its contents! So if you have any 'urgency' difficulties, it isn't a good idea to drink more than 1-2 cups of strong peppermint tea per day.

In fact, it is better to go for variety anyway. Try different teas and combinations, don't rely too consistently on one kind.

Chamomile is a good one to try. It's wonderful herb. It isn't just a marvelous relaxant, it is quite a powerful anti-inflammatory too, so if your sleep is disturbed due to pain it could help that. Don't chug it back like a drug though. Savor it, let it wash over your taste-buds and under your tongue (substances are absorbed more quickly into your bloodstream under the tongue).

It is said that if you try something 10 times you can develop a taste for it, even if you disliked it on first taste. That was certainly true for me with chamomile. I hated it at first - I thought it tasted like grass - but now I really love it and look forward to enjoying it as part of my bedtime ritual. If you really don't like it, try it with other herbs that you do like, so you get the taste for it. A little honey can help too.

My other favorites are:

- ➢ Nettle (full of iron)
- ➢ Rosehip (bursting with vitamin C)
- ➢ Fennel & cardamom (particularly good after a meal, as a digestive)
- ➢ Any blends containing hops or valerian.

If you don't like herbal tea, try brewing some and leaving it to go cold. The flavor can be less intense. I know parents who keep a jug of cold herbal tea out for their children during the summer months. They guzzle it happily without realizing what it is.

I'm not a huge fan of fruit teas as their ingredients often contain things that don't occur naturally - extractions, flavorings, etc.

## Daylight Lamps & Blackout Curtains

Getting your wake-sleep balance right can be helped by using a daylight lamp during the day and having blackout curtains or blinds in your bedroom. This is especially useful if you work shifts.

You can buy medically-approved daylight lamps for treating Seasonal Affective Disorder - a type of depression which descends during the darker months. I have one and use it from October to March. It sits on the desk where I write and I turn it on, generally, around midday for a few hours.

It is also possible to buy daylight bulbs for other household or office light fittings. They are known as full-spectrum bulbs or tubes. Buy as many as you can afford for areas where you spend a lot of time during the day.

Don't want to use them at night, as they could keep you awake. One solution to this is to have the full-spectrum bulbs in your main overhead light fittings and use more muted bulbs in smaller lamps to use during the evenings.

A lot of people suffer from insomnia and tiredness due to their habit of checking their emails and texts, surfing the Internet and watching television at night. These devices project unnatural light at times when you body is telling you to wind down for sleep. The light can disturb the body's natural rhythms - known as the circadian rhythms - and cause insomnia, fatigue, mood problems, etc. That is why a lot of sleep experts tell people to keep televisions out of bedrooms and avoid stimulating activities before bed.

We have lost our connection with nature. I keep hens and, summer or winter, they go to bed as dusk falls. That can be 4pm in winter and 10pm in summer. They don't care about the time, they just know that it's getting to sleepy time. They are NEVER tired next morning, they are always up with the sun, raring to go.

It is hard for modern humans to go back to nature and sleep when dusk falls though. We lead busy lives, we have jobs that often go on until after dark, and we have social lives.

One thing that works for me is a free piece of software called *F.lux*. It is available for Macs and Windows systems but unfortunately not for iPhones/iPads (yet, hopefully some clever programmers are working on it).

The people at *F.lux* have done their research and say that:

> *'An average person reading on a tablet for a couple of hours before bed may find that their sleep is delayed by about an hour'.*

They quote numerous scientific papers[13] which demonstrate that exposure to artificial light - in particular the blue light that computers and other devices emit - affects sleep. They say that using their software, which changes the color and intensity of the light emitted by a computer screen, lowers central nervous system activity, thereby encouraging natural, better sleep and relaxation.

As *F.lux* is free, it is certainly worth trying it out to see if it helps your quality of sleep.

## 2. REBOUNDING

Rebounding is trampolining for grown-ups. It gives us the chance to jump for joy and not be embarrassed about it! These little trampolines are such fun and provide an amazing and highly effective form of exercise.

I first read about them in the early 1980's, just after NASA had made a statement about the effects of rebounding:

---

[13] http://justgetflux.com/research.html

> *'... For similar levels of heart rate and oxygen consumption, the magnitude of the biomechanics stimuli is greater with jumping on a trampoline than with running.'*

The reason NASA had investigated rebounding was because of the deconditioning caused in astronauts by weightlessness. The deconditioning is similar to that experienced by people who have had extended bed rest. NASA found that rebounding helped their astronauts to avoid the health problems and they recommend it as an extremely effective form of exercise.

Even the esteemed Journal of Cardiopulmonary Rehabilitation shouted about the benefits of rebounding:

> *'The mini trampoline (rebounder) provides a convenient form of exercise with a major advantage being its apparent low level of trauma to the musculoskeletal system.'*
>
> (Journal of Cardiopulmonary Rehabilitation, 1990: 10; 401-408)

I tried it out and was amazed to find that even with my shattered ankles I could manage gentle rebounding - very gentle, not jumping, just a slight bounce by flexing the knees. Even this limited exercise is very effective because of the effect of gravity.

When you bounce up you achieve a weightless state and when you bounce down you experience twice the usual force of gravity. This means that every cell in your body is being exercised.

Rebounding, like skin brushing, also has a marked effect on the lymphatic system, increasing lymph flow in some cases by as much as 15 to 30 times.

There are numerous DVDs available, as well as free YouTube videos on how to rebound.

Here's my advice:

> ➢ Buy the best rebounder you can afford – a good used one is better than a 'cheap' new one. I started with an inexpensive new rebounder then bought a better quality used one from Ebay. It had hardly been used and I'm still enjoying it three years later. The difference between the cheap one and the more expensive one is massive. It is much easier and more pleasant to bounce on the more expensive one.

> ➢ Don't be tempted to jump on and do 20 minutes straightaway. Start with just a couple of minutes a day for the first week or so before building up gradually.

> ➢ Begin with the gentle bounce at first, not leaving the surface, just flexing your knees to achieve a nice up and down movement.

> ➢ Gradually start making the bounce bigger, until you start to leave the surface. Keep your knees soft and don't try to jump, just bounce.

You can then progress to more fancy moves, including star jumps, jogging and twists. I avoid twists because of back problems but you may find them okay for you.

People in wheelchairs can benefit from the effects of rebounding. When you have a physical disability it is really frustrating to read that we should all be taking more exercise and walking more. Well more than frustrating actually, it's discriminatory.

Yes, we do need to move to be healthy and if you are incapable of moving you will need to find some sort of passive exercise that you can do. You can sit with just your feet on a rebounder, while someone else bounces on it. The energy waves travel through your feet, stimulating the nerve endings and affecting the whole body.

This is a wonderful way to occupy children! The children feel they are doing a great service to you - as indeed they are. I had to do this for a while when my ankles were going through a really bad stage. My daughter was about 8 at the time and loved helping by bouncing me. It was fun too! The passive bouncing, combined with some skin brushing, was enough to keep my lymph glands in check while I was unable to walk for six months.

I can only manage a few minutes on a rebounder due to the pain in my ankles, but for those without mobility problems, a 20-minute session is fun and easy to do. I feel great benefits from just the few minutes I can manage though. It doesn't feel like exercise, it's more like play!

Here are a few links to articles that talk about rebounding. I like to read things like this when I feel a bit lazy and need some motivation. Reading about the benefits of rebounding makes you want to jump right on one!

**https://rebound-air.com/best_rebounding_33_ways.htm**

**http://blog.radiantlifecatalog.com/bid/57710/ Rebounding-Revisited-20-surprising-rebounder-benefits**

## 3. WATER & HYDROTHERAPY

After my accident I was stuck on a hospital ward for a week before being able to use a bathroom (I had a catheter!). I can still remember - 20+ years later - the wonderful feeling when I was able to get out of bed for the first time and asked to be taken to the bathroom to a tap just to feel cool water splooshing over my hands.

Most of us in first world countries, unaffected by water shortages, fail to appreciate water as much as we perhaps should.

Water therapy was used by the famous health clinics of the late 19th and early 20th centuries, such as Gerson, Bircher-Benner & Kellogg. They had expensive equipment but actually if you have a bathroom you have equipment that can replicate some of theirs.

1. Alternating **hot and cold showers**. Not as horrendous as it sounds! Have a hot shower for a few minutes, then switch to cool for 20-30 seconds; then hot again for a few more minutes; and cooler for up to 30 seconds. This zips up the circulation and makes you feel really quite invigorated. Cold water is also beneficial for the hair – particularly for frizz-prone types.

2. **Compresses**. A towel dipped in hot water and wrung out can help respiratory problems when applied to the chest. For safety, put the towel over a sheet or thin towel on your chest, so there's no danger of burning. Hot compresses can also be used for muscle pain and some joint pains. Cold compresses are better for certain arthritic pain – if you suffer you'll probably know whether hot or cold is better for you.

3. Alternating **hot and cold compresses**. These are good for sprains. I use them a lot on my ankles. Have a few minutes of heat followed by 30 seconds of cold, alternated a few times.

4. **Body wrap** or wet sheet pack. This was used by the naturopaths of old for cases of fever. The wet sheet needs to be dipped in cold (yes, really!) water. Wrap the person up in that and then wrap a nice warm blanket or fleece over that. The body heat dries the sheet, transferring wastes and toxins to it (to wash it before using it again, even on the same person).

5. **Salt scrubs**. These are good to do at the change of seasons, using an appropriate oil. Simply put 2 cups of sea salt in a bowl and drizzle 1½ cups of grapeseed oil over it. Then add 5-10 drops of the essential oil of your choice. Mix them together and get in the bath tub. Dip a wet hand in the bowl and rub the salt mix between your palms, then rub it all over your body. You want a scrubbing motion for this. It will feel very tingly. It is best done right at the end of a shower. Wash the salt mixture off after you've rubbed it all over your body (avoiding the eyes, nose, and any cuts/abrasions).
Good oils to choose from are:
   - ➢ Lemon.
   - ➢ Lime.
   - ➢ Grapefruit.
   - ➢ Rose.
   - ➢ Bergamot.
   - ➢ Peppermint.
   - ➢ Tea tree – mixed half and half with another oil if you don't like the smell.

6. **Hot & Cool Sitz baths**. These are very useful for pain in the pelvic area, including IBS. They can be difficult to do at home due to the practicalities but if you happen to have a baby bath large enough to sit in, you can use that and an

ordinary bath tub. Fill one with warm water and the other with cool water. Spend a few minutes sitting in the warm tub followed by 10-30 seconds sitting in the cool tub, then back to the warm tub. Repeat the cycle until it brings comfort – which it does, quite quickly.

# 4. EPSOM SALT BATHS & FOOTBATHS

Epsom Salts are known as a laxative, but they are also a powerful source of magnesium, which many people are deficient in. It is absorbed very well through the skin, so Epsom Salt baths and footbaths are an easy and inexpensive way to get magnesium into your body.

Magnesium deficiency is very common. Taking it in via the skin in this way avoids any concerns about excess that you might have if you took magnesium orally.

My fiancé suffers from Restless Legs Syndrome. It sounds a minor complaint but it can destroy your life by interrupting sleep and leaving you a walking zombie during the day. It doesn't leave your partner in a good mood either, if they share your bed!

Epsom Salt baths/footbaths are a good help for RLS and you can also make a spray solution (50/50 Epsom salts, dissolved in warm water and put into a spray bottle) to spray on your legs before bed if you don't have time to soak.

I buy my Epsom Salts in bulk online because we go through a lot. I take Epsom Salt baths twice a week, using 2 double handfuls of the salts in a hottish bath. You need to soak for 20 minutes to get the full effect, and also rub a bar of good soap through your hands under the water when you first submerge. The soap helps the absorption of the magnesium.

Choose an Epsom Salt bath/footbath - or even hand bath if you have painful hands - if you:

➢ Have been exercising. It reduces next-day muscle soreness.

➢ Suffer from arthritis or rheumatic-type pain of the joints.

➢ Suffer from Chronic Fatigue Syndrome or Fibromyalgia. It helps the muscle and joint pain.

➢ Know you are deficient in magnesium.

**NOTE**: Having a hot therapeutic bath is lovely but it isn't a good idea to make a hot bath a daily habit. It can be very debilitating. Naturopath Dr. Ross Trattler says in his book *Better Health through Natural Healing*:

> *"Very hot full-immersion baths daily create debility, poor circulation, mental lethargy, physical weakness, and depression."*

For this reason, it is best not to have the bath water too hot, not to stay in it longer than 20 minutes - unless you get out and splash yourself down with cold water, before getting back in for another 20 minute soak - and not have this sort of bath more than twice a week.

Showers are much more refreshing, especially if you have a tendency towards fatigue, poor circulation, and/or depression.

## 5. Tips For Beating Pain & Tension

We often experience pain as a result of tension in our bodies. If we can use a few tricks to reduce the tension, we can avoid the pain completely.

## The 2 Tennis Balls & A Sock Trick For Tension

This may sound odd, but has been recommended to me by several alternative health professionals and it really works. It is also mentioned in *Spent*, the wonderful health book by Dr Frank Lipman.

Put 2 tennis balls into the toe of a sock and tie a knot in the leg of the sock so that the tennis balls are held close together.

Lie down on the floor - on a rug, squishy towel, or mat if it is a hard floor - and place the sock under your neck, with a ball either side of your spine. The tennis balls should be applying slight pressure to the muscles of your neck, not the bones.

Lie still and relax, letting the tennis balls do their work on your muscles. We hold a lot of tension in our neck muscles and this is a fabulous method of releasing that.

If you have neck pain and don't have any tennis balls, try...

## The 2 Pillows & A Scarf Trick For Neck Pain

When I gave birth to my son I threw my neck out of joint with all the pushing. I was in horrible pain the next day and couldn't get any relief. My husband rang an osteopath, who gave over-the-phone advice which took away the pain immediately.

She told us to get a scarf and tie it tightly around the middle of a pillow. It makes the pillow look a little like a big puffy bow! Then put that pillow on top of another pillow and put both in a pillow case.

Lie down with the pillows under your neck and head. You need to have the knotted part of the top pillow directly under your neck.

This brings wonderful relief - very quickly - if you have neck pain caused by holding your head too far forward. This happens to a lot of computer users. People I massage also suffer from it and it seems to be caused by smartphone and tablet use - Kindles too. We tend to hold our necks at weird angles when using them.

Of course, if you have any serious damage to your neck, don't use either the tennis ball or knotted pillow techniques without advice from your doctor or specialist health professional. Really, you don't want to mess with your neck.

## The Reset Your Shoulders Trick For Tension In The Upper Back & Neck

This was taught to me by my fiancé, who learned it from his friend, a chiropractor.

- ➤ Find a door that has a sturdy frame. You want one that extends from the wall slightly, so you can stand underneath and put a hand each side, holding on to the top of the frame with your fingertips.
- ➤ Stand sideways in the doorway (this will cause strange stares if you have curious family members wandering in and out. Just smile. You're giving them free entertainment.).
- ➤ Let your fingertips take the weight of your upper body by relaxing your legs a little. You need to keep your feet on the floor, this isn't an endurance test, all you are doing is letting your arms take some of your weight. Your shoulders may protest a little because they have to move into the correct position to take your weight.

➢ Now move away from the door and circle your shoulders once to the front and once to the back.

➢ Raise your arms out to the sides and up above your head, then glide them down to your sides. Your shoulders should be further back than they were.

If you perform this exercise daily you will find they should stop being rounded forwards.

If you have problems, though, do go to a trained osteopath or chiropractor. They can do wonders for this sort of thing.

## Static Back Press For Back Pain

You know the way you can find treasure in the oddest of places? I did on vacation in Yorkshire. We came across a little used book store and I found a book by Pete Egoscue that has helped me tremendously. It made me understand why I suffer hip pain even though it's my ankles that were injured; why my knees started to get sore; and why my feet used to stick out to the sides.

Both his publisher and the famous golfer Jack Nicklaus describe Pete as an 'Anatomical Functionalist' but it would be more accurate to call him an anatomical genius. He just calls himself 'The Posture Guy'. His clinics (25 of them world-wide) are considered world leaders in non medical pain relief.

Pete has a knowledge of the human body that is incredible and devises exercises to get people back to full function. He has helped athletes, ex Presidents, and thousands of other people get back their health by improving their posture.

Static back press is one of his favorite exercises for reducing back pain. It is a simple, easy exercise that can be done almost anywhere.

> ➤ Lie on the floor with your calves resting on a coffee table or something similar. You want your thighs to be vertical and your calves parallel with the floor. My coffee table is ideal but before we got it I used to use a foam block.

> ➤ Put your arms out to the side with the palms up.

> ➤ Relax.

> ➤ Keep relaxing until your back pain goes. This can be just minute or two for some people, 20 minutes or more for others. In this position, your tense back muscles have no need to clench and are able to relax fully.

If you try static back press and like it, you might like to check out Pete's books and DVDs or - if you have health problems - see if you can get to one of his clinics.

I use his 'Pain Free Workout Series' DVD every day. Check out his website at:

**www.egoscue.com**

# 6. GET YOUR CIRCADIAN RHYTHMS IN SYNC

Circadian rhythms aren't some new dance move, but the inner biological processes of your body. One of the ways they can be disrupted is through bright lights at night. Your body naturally starts feeling sleepy as night closes in. We are programmed to sleep at night and be awake during daylight hours. If we disrupt those processes by using artificially bright lights to keep us alert at night, we mess with our sleep cycle. Having a bright light on when you should be winding down for bed is a bad idea; but most of us do it. We use computers into the small hours of the morning, we watch TV late, telling ourselves that it helps us sleep. Sorry, it doesn't. It probably helps you relax, but that's not the same as sleep. Here are some ideas for helping get your sleepy circadian rhythms back in their groove:

Turn down the lights at 10pm and turn off computers and TVs as soon after 10pm as you can get away with in your family. It may be best to do it gradually, over the course of a week or so. If your normal bedtime is midnight, turn the lights down at 11 and switch off the TV/computer at 11:30. Reading or listening to music before bed is much better for your brain and sleep cycle than watching TV.

I speak as a former addict. I HAD to watch a comedy before bed or I couldn't sleep. I like to go to sleep in a good mood, so it had to be a comedy. Then I read that sleep is really important and lack of sleep can inhibit weight loss. That was enough information to make me take action!

So I read up on it and discovered circadian rhythms. Once I learned about the importance of them in adopting healthy sleep habits, I was able to give up my late-night TV and switched to an MP3 player that allows me to put comedy videos on it. I barely hear the first 10 minutes before I'm asleep. The lack of flickering light has really helped my sleep. And my weight!

Those of us who work long hours at a computer will know how easy it is to keep on working and suddenly realize it has gone very dark outside. It's common for people working on computers to get eye, neck, and shoulder strain from overworking and hunching at a computer.

# 7. TRY A HERBAL ADAPTOGEN

If you need an energy boost, it's very tempting to reach for either caffeine or a sugary snack/drink. Some people need a salty snack if their adrenals are used to working overtime due to chronic stress. We put our bodies under additional stress when we habitually take these food stimulants, though. Once in a while is fine but if you rely on a coffee to get you going every morning, a sweet snack to get you through the mid afternoon energy slump, and sodas to keep your energy levels up, you are putting your body into a state of crisis.

If this is you, you might like to consider trying a herbal adaptogen. Adaptogens are clever - they boost you when you're sluggish and calm you down when you are hyper. Herbal manufacturers have been allowed since 1998 to claim the term 'adaptogen' as a function claim. Adaptogens have a physiological effect but there is also a placebo thing going on when you are taking them. You know you are taking something that is giving you more energy (if you don't have enough energy), so you feel you can do more.

I was able to come off a 5-year sleeping tablet habit addiction by taking herbal adaptogens. They gave me more energy during the day so I was able to be busy and get naturally tired. I combined this with gradually reducing my caffeine intake and taking Valerian tincture before bed to help me relax.

Scientific studies have shown that they work by affecting the sympathetic nervous system, having a soothing effect and protecting it from the negative effects of stress. One of the interesting things they do is protect against the bad effects of cortisol. Cortisol is raised when we are stressed and it can cause anxiety, irritability, weight gain, bone loss, and lethargy (among other things). Having something in our armory to bop cortisol on the head is wonderful!

Every continent seems to have its own adaptogen - Siberian ginseng, Indian Ashwaganda, Chinese astragalus, etc.

Adaptogens include:

> ➤ Siberian Ginseng - probably the best-known, thanks to its use by Russian scientists. Increases mental alertness, enhances athletic performance. Not just grown in Russia!

> ➤ Asian (Panax) Ginseng - acts as a tonic, helps the body & mind withstand stress, improves endurance. One study showed that it can counteract adrenal gland shrinkage

> ➤ Ashwaganda - eases anxiety, helps the immune system, and lowers cortisol levels.

> ➤ Licorice - increases endurance and energy, boosts the immune system, protects again cortisol damage. It has the huge benefit of being inexpensive too. Buy from herbal suppliers, not the candy shelves! NOTE: Don't use licorice without medical supervision if you have or could have high blood pressure.

> ➤ Astragalus - boosts immunity, helps repair and prevent damage caused by cortisol and other stress problems.

> ➤ Rhodiola - helps both mental and physical fatigue (used by Russian soldiers), reduces anxiety, may reduce the effects of aging, can help regulate appetite, protects the heart and liver, increases the body's use of oxygen, can help in cases of memory problems. Rhodiola has been the subject of a lot of research and it has been linked to weight loss and longevity.

You can take adaptogens on their own or as part of a blend. They are generally considered safe, with the exception of licorice which can't be taken by people with high blood pressure. I have had wonderful blends made for me by medical herbalists. They take the time to find out more about your unique constitution and come up with powerful yet safe herbal prescriptions.

# 8. Natural Energy Boosters

I over-relied on diet colas for two years while running a business, believing that the caffeine in them gave me an energy boost. Well it probably did, at the beginning, but I had to drink more and more cola to get the effect I wanted and that caused weight gain, sore teeth, and frayed nerves. I finally gave up when I started to suffer a racing heart and symptoms of anxiety. Now I use natural energy boosters, I'm amazed at how much more effective they are.

If you need a jolt of energy, it is much better to try natural energy boosters such as:

➢ An apple and a couple of almonds or a teaspoon of peanut butter.

➢ An apple and a small handful of sunflower seeds. Sunflower seeds are amazing little powerhouses. They're packed with nutrients (over 80!) and are a particularly good source of protein and essential fatty acids.

➢ A cup of ginseng tea.

➢ A cup of peppermint and licorice tea (if you don't have high blood pressure).

➢ A homemade juice containing a carrot, an apple, and a thumbnail-size piece of fresh ginger. Delicious, even for people who don't usually like juices that contain vegetables!

➢ Tyrosine, an amino acid that is a natural stimulant. It enters the brain quickly and can improve your mood and energy. It is even said to help cognitive ability and motivation. As always, check with your doctor to make sure that it won't interact with anything else you're taking.

➢ A couple of squares of dark chocolate instead of a whole bar of milk chocolate. This is what really helped get rid of my chocolate habit. Mostly because I didn't really like it! Not as much as milk chocolate anyway. I could honestly eat a 1lb bar of milk chocolate, but can't manage more than a couple of squares of dark chocolate.

➢ Get some sun. Even if you live in colder northern climates you will almost certainly have some sunlight most days - if not it will be pitch dark. Get outside at noon if you possibly can, even if only for 5 minutes.

➢ Try green tea. It gives the metabolism a mild boost.

➢ Do some stretches. We often get tired and apathetic when sitting or standing. Getting up for a quick walk around and doing a few stretches can get the circulation going, increase oxygen consumption, and make you feel much better.

➢ Do some deep breathing. Deep breathing not only brings in fresh oxygen, it improves lymphatic flow, helping the body get rid of the waste products that could leave you feeling sluggish.

➢ Drink some water. A lot of tiredness is caused by dehydration. Add some fresh lemon juice or greens powder for a potassium boost, to improve the hydrating effect on every cell in your body.

## Things To Consider Swapping Or Giving Up

It's best to add things to your diet and lifestyle before working on any things that you need to remove. That creates a feeling of abundance and nourishment and reduces the amount of stress you experience once you do start giving food, drink, or habits up.

When you feel ready you probably know what you need to work on: less alcohol, less processed foods, less dodgy fats, etc. The best way to go about giving those up is to do is gently, one at a time, and to substitute them for a healthier alternative.

Here are a few things to consider:

> We often crave things that aren't good for us. Sometimes we have an actual intolerance to them, or are addicted to them. If there's something you feel you can't do without – say alcohol, nicotine, drugs, or a particular food – then you might have a problem with that. Try tapering off gently and see how you go. If it is a problem you might find it easier with the help of a nutritionist, counselor, or other health professional. It isn't weak to accept help, it's smart. It is often quicker and less stressful to get the assistance of a professional who is used to coaching people through withdrawal.

> People who are trying to lose weight who keep a food journal have more success than those who don't. Keep a record of what you eat, drink, and do and you'll be able to spot patterns. There may be things that cause you to overindulge in some way – these are known as **trigger foods** but they aren't limited to foods. Alcohol is a well-known one, of course. Once you start drinking you lose your inhibitions and your self-control. There are others, though. Peanut butter is a trigger food for many people (me included!). Tim Ferriss phrased it brilliantly in *The Four-Hour Body*, after advising the consumption of a tablespoon of peanut butter to stave off hunger pangs before bed:

> *Note to the ladies, for whom peanut butter seems to be like crack: the tablespoon scoop should be no more than a small mound, not half the jar balanced on a spoon.*
>
> Tim Ferriss, *The Four-Hour Body*

➤ Food and drink aren't the only bad habits. You might be in the habit of over-exercising or not exercising enough (at all?!), negative thought patterns, lack of assertiveness, or routine anger. Keeping a journal can again help as you will be able to see your negative reactions. I got into the habit of keeping a thought journal after reading the book *Mind Over Mood*. It was immensely helpful. Within a week or two, I was able to recognize when my thoughts were about to head into a downward spiral and stop them.

## Healthy Food Swaps

Check out these websites for ideas of healthy food swaps:

**www.nhs.uk/Livewell/loseweight/ Pages/Healthyfoodswaps.aspx#close**

**www.womansday.com/health-fitness/ nutrition/50-Healthy-Food-Swaps**

**www.healthinsite.gov.au/article/ healthy-food-swaps**

In general, try to swap any food made in a factory for food made by smaller suppliers. Then food made by smaller suppliers for food made at home.

## MAKING CHANGES THAT STICK

It's one thing taking up a new habit with the first rush of enthusiasm, it's another keeping going, especially at 6 in the morning when you're rushed for work.

My friend Steve Scott runs a website devoted to the idea of developing good habits, one at a time. It's at:

**www.developgoodhabits.com/**

You can get [free] ideas and inspiration on there for new good habits to take up and ways to build your willpower muscle!

# CHAPTER 16
# BRUSHING MOTIVATION: 7 QUICK TIPS TO KEEP YOU BRUSHING

CR80

WHAT ABOUT DAYS when you feel too tired to feel like brushing? What about mornings when you get up late and are in a mad rush?

If you are like most people, a busy lifestyle and uncontrollable circumstances will combine to prevent you from brushing sometimes. The danger is that you'll feel like a failure and give up completely.

Let's put some strategies in place so that doesn't happen. Put at least two of these things in place right from Day One, then you'll be prepared for the unexpected.

1. If you are in a rush in the morning, take your brush to the bathroom and at least do a quick brush of your chest, neck, face, arms, hands, and torso. For me, this is best accomplished while perching on the edge of the bath or the

toilet seat (too much information alert – you can even brush while on the toilet, ultimate multi-tasking!).

2. Put your brush on the bathroom floor and brush your feet while cleaning your teeth. Hold it down by stepping on the handle with one foot while brushing the other.

3. If mornings are too busy or frantic, get in the habit of taking some 'me' time and brushing at some other point during the day. I prefer to brush in the mornings because, frankly, I need the extra energy it gives me. Sometimes, though, the dog has been sick or my daughter is late for work or my son needs me to run him somewhere and I just don't get chance to brush. On those days, I'll choose to have an early bath that evening. Brushing before the bath helps my skin to absorb any goodies I put into the bath (such as the Epsom Salts baths I mentioned earlier).

4. Adopt the super fast brushing routine that you can do in 60 seconds. Most people can spare 60 seconds even when in a hurry. Brush each section just once and you should find that you can cover your entire body in under a minute.

5. Write out some of the points from this book that 'spoke' to you - the reasons that you are doing skin brushing. Stick up the piece of paper somewhere obvious - I have mine inside my wardrobe door so I read them when I open it. It's a good reminder in case I start to get dressed without brushing first! Some people prefer a Post-It note on the bathroom mirror. You may find that a reminder like this is very motivating. Keeping the benefits of skin brushing to mind will help you keep up the momentum.

6. Make a note of improvements in your skin, tone, energy, and any other wonderful bonuses, as they happen. It is easy to forget how you used to feel, and writing them down

is very motivating. Read them back whenever you need a nudge to get you to pick your brush up.

7. Take your body measurements. If you need to tone up anywhere, you should notice improvements very quickly when you start skin brushing. Thighs are often the first to start toning up, which is really encouraging, as they can be quite hard to tone otherwise. You may also notice a difference in the bingo wing area (upper arms) and saddlebag area (the hips). The waist area can also noticeably improve within a few days of starting skin brushing.

# CHAPTER 17
# EXCUSES EXCUSES

CRRO

**I**T IS HUMAN nature to start a new project with great hope and enthusiasm, and then give it up once the initial burst of energy which accompanies something new wears off.

Being aware of this possibility is good because you can guard against it.

Here are some ~~excuses~~ reasons you might have to deal with from your inner rebel - forewarned is forearmed.

## IT'S TOO COLD WHERE I LIVE

I hear you. I live in the north of England and Russia is only a bit further north than us. It is often too cold to want to spend any length of time without clothes on.

However, being too cold to skin brush is an excellent reason to take up skin brushing because there's nothing quite like it for getting warm.

Brushing your skin brings the blood rushing to the surface. After a few minutes of brushing, your skin with be buzzing and warm, and you will feel a glorious rush of energy as well that will keep you going all morning.

Knowing that makes it easier to take your clothes off. If it is dangerously cold, though, just try exposing and brushing one body part at a time.

## IT'S TOO HOT WHERE I LIVE

The good thing about this is that you won't mind at all being without clothes! You won't want to stimulate your circulation too much though.

The way to cope with that is to refrain from brushing vigorously. If you brush slowly and gently you won't get the same warmth in your skin as you do if you brush firmly and quickly.

Follow the brushing with a cool shower and you will soon cool down.

If you need the effects of stimulating your circulation, though, you may want to get up early - before the sun is fully risen - to do your skin brushing, and take a nap later on.

## MY MOBILITY IS LIMITED

There are ways round this. You can:

> Just brush the parts you can reach. You will get benefits from just brushing your face and neck.

> Get someone else to brush you. This doesn't have to be embarrassing, you could wear a swimsuit. The main clusters of lymph glands that you want to reach are in the groin (so brushing the legs is great), armpits (brushing up

the arms and down from the neck gets to these), and neck (brush the face and head).

➢ If you can't reach your feet but can move them, use your brush bristles-up on the floor, perhaps resting against something, and move your feet over the brush.

➢ Try a change of position. Some people struggle to bend down towards their feet but can reach them (using the brush handle) if they put their legs straight out on a bed. This is helpful if you have high blood pressure, balance problems, middle ear problems, and other things that make you go woozy if you bend down. I went through a period of this - never found out what it was, but I fainted if I bent down low (it only lasted a few weeks). I got around it by propping my foot up on my dresser when I brushed - it is higher than the bed so didn't give me that horrible dizziness.

Brushing could help to improve your mobility a little, it is like a gentle form of exercise in itself.

## I DON'T HAVE TIME TO BRUSH IN THE MORNINGS BEFORE I SHOWER

That's fine. You can brush after your shower, or when you get home from work, perhaps when changing your clothes.

The idea of brushing before a shower is so you can wash away any dead skin cells that you brushed but haven't fallen off yet. It isn't a biggie though as you will be showering next morning anyway and, after a short time, you will have brushed off the backlog of cells that had built up on your skin and you will only be brushing away a very small amount each time.

I often brush at night, when I'm more relaxed and have more time. If you are brushing right before bed, don't be too vigorous. A quick morning brush is a great way to start the day but there's nothing like a longer, more luxurious brushing when you have more time. Try to see it as a type of massage that you can do yourself. Keep the strokes slow and pampering and you won't over-stimulate yourself before sleep.

## I CAN'T AFFORD A GOOD BRUSH

I hear you. We've been through some difficult financial times as a family and I know what it is like to be unable to buy even little things for yourself. For Moms especially, we will buy things for our children but not for ourselves. For two years I didn't have a cup of coffee at home because of the expense of boiling the kettle but I made sure my children were able to go to the movies with their friends.

I wish I could come round and give you a hug and a beautiful new brush. It's horrible being so short of money, a constant stress. You don't need me doling out silly advice about budgeting, selling things on Ebay, or giving up something else so you can afford a brush.

One thing I would say, though, is this: if you don't make your own health a priority, you aren't going to be on top form to be there for your family. It's that oxygen mask thing again!

If you can't afford a brush because you spend on your children - or animals, or other family members/friends/strangers in the street - then maybe you could explain to your loved ones that this is something you'd really like, that would make you feel healthier and happier, and that you'd love their support in being able to buy. Children can be very enterprising when it comes to making money! Maybe they'll set up a lemonade stand to raise the funds. Well in many areas that isn't safe anymore, unfortunately, but they may be good on computers and will know a few places to sell things. Allowing them to help you is not only teaching them good life skills, it's giving them an opportunity to give back, which is good for the soul and the ego.

If all else fails and you can't raise any funds for a good brush, then don't give up entirely. Get a cheap brush, if you can, in a store such as Walmart. They regularly have a brush for under $5. It is quite soft-bristled but it will do as a starter brush and you'll find it fine for your face and neck.

If you can't find/afford one, then use your hands, try a washcloth, anything, just get that lymph moving. I tried just using my hands instead of my brush for a few days and my skin was still much softer than not doing any movements.

Do aim to get your own good brush when you can though. Birthdays and Christmas are good times for dropping firm hints!

## I DON'T HAVE ANY PRIVACY AND MY BATHROOM IS TOO SMALL

You do need privacy for an all-over body brushing. I always felt that I had no privacy when my children were small. Here are a few ideas:

> ➤ Get up 10 minutes earlier than everyone else and do your brushing as soon as you wake.

> ➤ Tell the family/rest of the household that you need 20 minutes to yourself when you get home from work (or when another caregiver in the house gets home from

work). Use this time to brush, take a quick shower, and just spend some quiet 'me' time.

➢ Try brushing in the bathroom anyway. My bathroom is small and my mobility is limited so I prefer to brush in my bedroom, where I can sit on the bed and prop my foot on a bookcase for doing my legs. I can, however, manage to do my brushing by sitting on the edge of the tub for the upper part of my body and propping my foot on the toilet for my legs. Not ideal and not very comfortable but adequate.

➢ Brush in the shower itself, before switching on the water. If you can't reach your feet/legs in the shower, don't worry, just do your upper half, trunk, and hips/butt. Treat your legs later on by resting with them propped up on a wall.

## I TRIED IT YEARS AGO BUT GOT OUT OF THE HABIT

➢ You can get back in the habit by doing this 10-day plan. 10 days are enough to convince yourself of the amazing benefits that skin brushing brings. 10 days are also enough to create the brain and muscle memories that go towards establishing a new habit. We're very much creatures of habit and if you can keep up your brushing for a few days, at least, you are on the way to creating a habit that you will actually find hard to break.

➢ Using my method brings great benefits in terms of lymphatic system stimulation, so you will experience better results than you may have done in the past. That in itself is very motivating. You want to continue to see what else improves!

> ➢ You could try scheduling time to do your skin brushing. Actually adding it to your calendar/diary/to do list can really help but only if you're not going to beat yourself up if you skip a session! Don't add skin brushing as yet another stressor, just fit it in when you can as a way of looking after yourself for a change.

> ➢ According to G.J. Fogg, PhD, a social scientist and behavior researcher at Stanford University, habits that we start doing in the mornings or evenings work more effectively than, say, ones we add in the middle of the day.

> ➢ Finally, don't worry about keeping up the skin brushing routine every single day after the first 10 days. The 10 days are necessary to exfoliate your skin, free up your pores, stimulate your blood and lymph flow, and help your other overworked elimination organs. The initial boost will sustain you so that you can just keep it topped up by brushing on weekends, when you have a bit more time for self-care.

# CHAPTER 18
## SPECIFIC PROBLEM AREAS

CʒᏠᎷᎾᏅ

WHOLE BODY BRUSHING is great but there may be areas you can't brush and many people have problem areas that they want to concentrate on for added benefits. That's fine.

Listed here are areas to avoid and areas where you might want to do extra brushing, and perhaps some massage.

## AREAS TO AVOID & WHY

There are problems that mean you shouldn't do any sort of massage - including skin brushing. These are listed in *Appendix 1 Contraindications For Skin Brushing*. There are also certain parts of the body you will need to avoid:

☒ Don't brush over any cuts, bruises or swellings - including acne. Brushing can help acne by stimulating the lymphatic system generally, but it won't help if you spread the acne with the brush.

☒ Don't brush over or anywhere near any varicose veins. You'll know if you have them, they will be swollen and/or painful. Generally they are to be found on the backs of the legs but they can be on other areas of the body. It is fine to brush above and below but avoid any areas near swollen, knotted veins completely. The pain isn't worth it and the brush could damage the veins and cause even more problems.

You **can** brush the face, neck and décolletage but if you have sensitive or thin skin be very careful and perhaps use a second, softer brush. If even a soft brush is too harsh, you can get similar benefits from using the same movements with your hands or a cloth. I have sensitive skin and am able to brush my face now but with very gentle brush strokes. I find it gives me a healthy glow but I do stress that it needs to be very gentle. The décolletage is an area that does benefit from brushing. It can quickly look aged, as the skin is so thin, and as skin brushing can help with the production of collagen, it is exactly what you need. Again, try a soft brush.

Don't brush any areas of the body which have lymphedema - swelling of the tissues caused by a buildup of lymphatic fluid. This is common after cancer treatment and requires very specialist treatment. If you can afford it, manual lymphatic drainage, a specialized form of massage, can bring massive relief.

Be very careful with the hands and feet if you suffer from Raynaud's disease/syndrome. People with Raynaud's have extremely cold hands and/or feet, caused by impaired blood flow. They can be so cold that they become discolored. It can be idiopathic (without a known cause) or be due to a connective tissue disorder. Lupus is one cause. It is often triggered or made worse by stress and cold. The temptation is to get your hands/feet warm by any means and brushing could seem a good way. It is important, though, to get medical advice first. Massage and brushing may be fine but it is best to check with an expert before jumping in. If you are given the OK, start with massage and move onto gentle brushing once you are used to the massage and responding well to it.

If in doubt about any part of your body, don't brush. Check with a doctor or other health practitioner first. You can get excellent benefits by just brushing the rest of your body and leaving out troublesome parts.

## AREAS TO CONCENTRATE ON & WHY

One way of concentrating on problem areas is to do an all-body brushing but use more strokes on the problem area(s). For instance, my inner thighs aren't as tight as I'd like them so, when I'm doing my luxurious weekend brushing sessions, on my thighs I will start with the inner section, do the other three sections, then the inner section again. You may have different areas you want to concentrate on. Here are a few examples:

### *Abdomen - Constipation*

If you have constipation or a sluggish bowel, you should see some improvement when you start brushing. Don't go at it too vigorously but if you have an episode of constipation, brush your abdomen a little more than usual. Use slow brush strokes - don't stress your bowel - and go in the direction of peristalsis (the natural movements of the bowel), which is clockwise. Start the brush on your lower abdomen by your right hip, brush up towards your waist a few times, then across your waist (passing over your belly button) a few times, then down the left side of your abdomen from around your left hip towards your groin.

This can be very effective, especially if you combine it with increased water consumption. Constipation can be extremely uncomfortable and often downright painful. You feel like you've taken poison, completely wretched.

When I had had an operation, years ago, one of the ladies on my ward had had a hysterectomy (removal of the uterus) a few days previously. She was in awful pain and groaned constantly. I asked one of the nurses if hysterectomies always caused such pain and was astonished to learn that the pain wasn't the result of the surgery, it was caused by constipation and trapped wind. The poor lady had become constipated due to inactivity following the surgery and because she wasn't drinking enough water.

I started to take drinking water and daily exercise a lot more seriously after that. She really was in a lot of pain.

The movement of the brush is similar to taking exercise, it gets the blood and lymph flowing in the region of the abdomen. You can combine it with some gentle exercise as well, if you are able to. Squats are good, as is walking. Rebounding is particularly good.

An exercise that can bring quick relief to the pain of constipation is to lie on your back and raise your knees towards your chest hold them, if you can, with your arms, hugging them towards you. Stay in this position for as long as is comfortable. It can be very effective at expelling trapped gas (so do it alone!).

When brushing, be sure to brush in the right direction, which is up from the right hip on the right side, across towards the left hip, and down towards the groin on the left side. Start at the belly button with small circles and gradually make them bigger until you are covering your whole lower abdomen. Brush your abdomen - gently - several times a day if you have to.

The opposite of constipation is diarrhea. There are many causes but one surprising one is actually constipation. If you are 'blocked' then only fluid can get past the blockage. In this case brushing can be tried but it can be overly stimulating (you don't want griping) so be very gentle. Tender massaging movements with your hands - preferably using a drop of a soothing essential oil such as fennel in a little vegetable oil - would be safer.

In both cases, constipation and diarrhea, be sure to get medical advice rather than trying to self-medicate - which could make the problem chronic.

In the meantime, be diligent about keeping up your water intake as that can really help and, in the case of diarrhea, can even be a lifesaver.

---

### ESSENTIAL OILS FOR CONSTIPATION
*Ginger, fennel, rosemary, orange, marjoram, black pepper, basil.*

You will often see peppermint recommended for digestive problems but I would urge you to use it with caution if you think your bowel may be sluggish. Peppermint is a smooth muscle relaxer. If your bowel is relaxed enough, don't use peppermint.

It can be very soothing for an irritated, over-active bowel though.

---

## Thighs & Upper Arms - Cellulite

Most women know about cellulite, even trim and toned Princess Diana apparently had a little of it. It is the name for fatty deposits just below the surface of the skin. They appear to be bumpy or dimpled and usually affect the outside of the thighs and, in some people, the upper arms.

Some doctors deny its existence - these are MALE doctors! Women know for sure it exists, as do some men. Dr Eric Berg says that cellulite is caused by muscle atrophe, which explains why both massage and skin brushing can help or eliminate it, due to their effect on muscle tone. Skin brushing can get rid of cellulite completely in many cases.

You will need to be persistent with your daily brushing, concentrate on the thighs a little more than other body areas and keep up your increased water intake. I noticed a difference after just a week and my cellulite had completely disappeared within a month. Some people report that it takes a little longer - 2-3 months - but it will help and hopefully cure even the most stubborn cellulite.

## Anti-Cellulite Routine

Brush as normal but, when you get to your thighs, on the outer thighs double the number of brush strokes. When you have finished your whole body (it is important to do the whole body, not just the thighs), you can add to the benefits by finishing with some massage of your thighs, using a helpful oil. The oils in the box are good for cellulite, circulation, and fat dispersal. Use a combination of two or three, depending on your personal preference. For example, juniper is a wonderful oil for cellulite, being a diuretic, tonic, and digestive. However, many people (me included) dislike the smell. So blend it with another oil on the list that you do like the smell of - lemon or grapefruit are good choices.

---

### ESSENTIAL OILS FOR CELLULITE

Juniper, lemon, grapefruit, rosemary,
peppermint, ginger, geranium.

---

## Upper Arms & Armpits - Pain

The armpits contain big clusters of lymph glands and they can get congested, swollen, and painful. One way to help the pain is to drink more water. As we saw earlier, the nodes take a lot of water out of the lymph, making it slower and thicker. Drinking more keeps everything flowing better.

If your armpits are painful, encourage them to decongest by placing the flat of your hand across your armpit and using a gentle pressure inwards and upwards, about 30 times. Do this before brushing your arm.

Be sure to do some deep breathing as it is very effective at helping lymph flow.

When brushing, concentrate on brushing up the arms, over the shoulder, and towards the back of the neck. This gently encourages some of the lymph to go to the lymph glands at the back of the neck, rather than the armpit. Do this until the pain lessens.

All over brushing will improve lymph flow generally, as will deep breathing, exercise, and drinking water.

## Upper Arms – Bumpy Skin

Bumpy skin on the upper arms is known as keratosis pilaris. It can also appear on the thighs and/or bottom. The little raised lumps are often slightly red in color. It is distinct from cellulite because the bumps are smaller and rougher.

There are several causes. Nutritionists say keratosis pilaris is sometimes caused by lack of essential fatty acids in the diet. These are often deficient in modern diets - even more so because the 'good' fats are needed to process all the 'bad' fats we eat.

Many dietitians recommend adopting the so-called Mediterranean diet, rich in olive oil, fish, avocados, and other fresh produce. This sort of way of eating is wonderful for the skin, it thrives on the oil.

Keratosis pilaris can also be caused by malabsorption, when the body simply can't benefit from the nutrients it takes in, so becomes deficient in various nutrients. One cause of this is gluten intolerance. Far from being a new age fad, gluten intolerance is a widespread problem.

You may also want to consider a more exotic addition too. Coconut oil has amazing health properties. I take 3 tablespoons a day. It helped my weight-loss (although I still have a way to go there but I'm doing it healthily, so no sagging skin!), increased my energy, and did amazing things with my skin. I barely need moisturizer.

Finally, some keratosis pilaris is caused by ingrown hairs and/or inflammation of the hair follicles.

Whatever the reason, skin brushing can help because it removes the dead skin cells, smooths the skin, and increases blood and lymph flow to the area (bringing fresh oxygen and nutrients and taking away wastes).

Do increased brush strokes on the bumpy areas of your upper arms when doing your full body skin brushing. If you don't have time for a full session, then at least do your upper arms.

## Face & Neck - Acne

Of course you can't brush the acne itself but you can use your - very clean - hands to encourage lymphatic movement in the area. When Dr Emil Vodder was developing his manual lymphatic drainage technique, he regularly cured patients' acne just by getting the lymphatic flow moving.

The head and neck are packed with lymph glands and they are, fortunately, quite easy to work on. There are lymph gland clusters to the front and back of the ears, below the ears, under the chin and lower jaw, and at the side/front of the neck. Use the flats of your hands and fingers to encourage lymph flow here.

Start at the neck. The best position is to cross your hands - left hand working on the right/front side of your neck and right hand working on the left. Place your hands on the skin of your neck lightly and press down and slightly towards the center of your body gently. This is a slight movement but it is very significant as it opens up the initial lymph vessels and starts a pump and vacuum flow of lymph. Move the hands up slightly and repeat the process.

Do the same at the chin - crossed hands again. This needs smaller movements as the area is small. Work on and below the lower jawbone, from the center of the chin out towards the ears.

Then place your hands - uncrossed this time - on the sides of your face. On each side you need to have three fingers in front of your ear and one finger (your index finger) behind it. Same skin movement again, down and slightly in towards the center of your body.

While doing the massage, breathe deeply and luxuriously. Don't stress over this, it's a reassuring movement for your mind and body. Think of this as your 'me' time and enjoy it, knowing that it is going to help your acne very quickly.

Once the acne has cleared up, you can progress to using your brush very gently in the same areas that you massaged. This will stimulate repair of any acne scars.

This is a subject close to my heart because I suffered from acne as a teenager and so did my daughter. I know the emotional agony of loathing the face in the mirror. It goes on for years, too.

We both tried prescriptions and doctor support but they didn't help. Many prescriptions are too harsh for delicate complexions. They dry out the skin and leave it looking scaly and uncared for.

Here are some other things you can do to help acne which worked for us:

> Avoid chemical cleansers. Use a good natural cleanser or switch to using simple almond (or grapeseed) oil to cleanse your face. I know, it seems ridiculous to put oil on oily skin but it really helps. Oil dissolves oil and daily application will make the oil producing glands in your skin realize that they don't need to keep working so hard. Put a light film of oil over your face and neck and remove it with a freshly washed cloth (preferably muslin) which has been dipped in hot water and then wrung out. You may need to re-dip it a few times until all the oil has been removed. Let your skin dry naturally, don't rub it with a towel.

> You can make your own toner very inexpensively by combining white hazel with rosewater. Add a couple of drops of your favorite essential oil. Lavender is good, as are geranium, rose, lemon, and ylang-ylang.

➢ Use an oil-free moisturizer or serum, or make your own. Natural oils are great – I use almond oil – but not good under make-up, as it can slide off!

➢ Go without makeup whenever you can, use an oil-free foundation when you can't do without some coverage. Estee Lauder's Double Wear is excellent.

➢ Use a foundation brush to apply foundation and be sure to keep it clean. You can get brush cleanser that it simply sprayed on and wiped off on a tissue. Quick and easy.

➢ If you need a body moisturizer there's a great recipe for an easy whipped coconut body butter here:

**http://bit.ly/coconutbodybutter**

Sleep on a satin or silk pillow. Buy several, so you can change and wash them daily. We get them inexpensively from Ebay.

➢ Keep your hair off your face - it can transfer oil. If you have bangs, pin them up. I saw a cashier with a gorgeous hairstyle just the other day. She had plaited her bangs and pinned them under the sides of her hair. It looked natural and stylish.

➢ Try not to touch your face. Many of us have the habit of leaning on a table and resting out chin in our hand. That's one to break if you have acne.

➢ Drink water in preference to milk. Milk is fine for growing babies but not the best thing for acne. If you can, switch to a dairy-free milk for a while to see if it helps (you may need a calcium and magnesium supplement if you don't have any other good calcium foods in your diet such as leafy green vegetables, sesame seeds, or almonds).

➢ Be scrupulous about keeping any makeup brushes, pads, or other implements you use on your face very, very clean.

➢ Eat a good variety of fresh fruit and vegetables but not too much fruit. An apple a day is great but fruit at every meal can mean too much fruit sugar for an acne-prone system. Have a wide variety of vegetables and you'll be getting vitamins and minerals in their most natural, and easily digestible, form.

➢ Have some protein at every meal. In particular, don't eat carbs on their own. They cause a rise in insulin and destabilized blood sugar.

➢ Take supplements if you can afford good ones. A multi-nutrient daily is a good insurance policy, as is a B-complex.

➢ Avoid stress as much as possible. Remove yourself from aggravating situations rather than putting up with them and seething inside. Take up some relaxing hobbies such as swimming, Pilates, walking in the country, etc..

If all else fails and you can't get rid of your acne, see a holistic doctor or medical herbalist.

## Face & Neck - Aging

It may seem ridiculous to consider brushing the sensitive skin of the face but it can have tremendous benefits. Brushing helps collagen production, the stuff in your skin that acts as a support system. When collagen breaks down, with age, skin starts to look older and less firm. With enough collagen loss, you get sagging.

Skin brushing boosts collagen production by increasing blood and lymph circulation and bringing fresh blood, oxygen, and lymph to the skin, and by exfoliating (removing dead skin cells). Exfoliating makes the skin produce new cells, which also includes new collagen.

Contrary to what skin care product manufacturers would have us believe, there is not much benefit in putting moisturizers containing collagen on the skin. The molecules are generally too large to penetrate the skin's barrier and aren't the same as the collagen we naturally produce.

Other things that can naturally boost collagen include:

> Vitamin C from oranges, lemons, and green vegetables.

> Beans - which contain hyaluronic acid, an anti-aging substance that is in a lot of expensive moisturizers and anti-aging products.

> Add flaxseeds or flaxseed oil to your diet. It contains easily absorbable omega-3s, which plump up and strengthen your skin. I add flaxseeds to my morning smoothie or, ground, to cereal.

> Avoiding sunburn.

> Getting enough protein. Collagen is made from amino acids (building blocks of protein) so making sure you have enough protein in your diet is very important.

> Using a good, natural moisturizer daily. Use one with a sunblock if you live in a hot climate and/or spend a lot of time outdoors. I use simple coconut oil as a moisturizer, it is inexpensive, pure, and very effective.

> Avoid smoky atmosphere (or give up smoking, if you smoke). Smokers have noticeably older looking skin than non-smokers. It contributes to the breakdown of existing collagen and reduces the body's ability to make new collagen.

# CHAPTER 19
# RESOURCES & SOURCES

☙❧

## BOOKS

### Zoe Harcombe's books

Zoe is the renowned UK nutritionist who taught me about the Minnesota Starvation Experiment and the fact that the human body needs 1,500 calories per day just for basic functioning.

Her books are no-nonsense, easy to read and understand, and packed with practical, affordable advice. Hers are the only 'diet' books I have come across that tackle the triple problems of Candida, food intolerance, and hypoglycaemia

### Dr Eric Berg's Books (and free YouTube videos)

Dr Berg is a Virginia-based chiropractor and health teacher who brings a breath of fresh air to the sometimes confusing world of health advice. His no-nonsense, practical suggestions make getting healthy fun and possible.

He has a YouTube channel packed with free videos and responds to comments on them. His books, *The 7 Principles of*

*Fat Burning* and *Adrenal Fatigue: Understanding the Symptoms of Adrenal Fatigue* are superb for anyone who has ever struggled to lose weight.

## Dr Frank Lipman's books

Dr Lipman achieved widespread attention when Gwyneth Paltrow consulted with him. That may be enough to put you off if you're anti New Age type stuff but actually he's a real doctor and gives sound advice. His book *Spent* is something I return to again and again, as is another of his books, *Revive*.

## Dr Daniel Amen's books

Dr Daniel Amen is a highly respected neuro-surgeon who embraces complementary medicines and healthy lifestyle changes. I love his theory about the 'ANTs' that destroy our health - Automatic Negative Thoughts.

He put forward the idea that our default position is negativity. It is part of our inbuilt survival skills to look out for potential dangers and possible disasters but it's now known that we tend to find what we are looking for. The brain looks for and recognizes patterns, it likes finding things it recognizes. So if you buy a red car, thinking that it's quite an unusual color and you don't see many red cars around - you'll be surprised to suddenly start noticing lots of red cars. It's because you're tuned into them and start noticing them.

Similarly, if you feel rejected by someone just once, you will be hyper-aware of the possibility of it happening again. You will start to look for it everywhere, from a dog not reacting to your inviting it to sniff your hand (when it was just recovering from an operation and still scared to move), to the postman missing out your house on his round (when actually there wasn't any post for you that day). You will then put up barriers, "I don't care anyway" or "Leave me alone, I couldn't cope with another rejection" barriers that make further perceived rejections more likely as people tend to avoid you because you give off vibes they don't quite understand.

Dealing with the automatic negative thoughts can make a huge difference to your health - and your job, your prospects, your income, your relationships, everything.

Dr Amen's books deal with a lot of practical issues surrounding brain health as well and aren't off-puttingly scientific. They can help you change your default position from negativity to positivity.

I highly recommend *Change your brain, change your life*, and *Change your brain, change your body*.

## OTHER HELPFUL THINGS

### *The Lightning Process*

**www.lightningprocess.com**

I couldn't miss this out as it was a big breakthrough for me on my own journey back to health. Phil Parker has combined his training in osteopathy, NLP (Neuro-Linguistic Programming), and life coaching to put together the most amazing system. It is mostly known for helping people with CFS, but can actually help people either deal with or get over a wide range of illnesses.

It enables you to break out of the cycle of living on adrenaline, feeling awful, crashing and needing an artificial boost to get going again.

I think completely well people should do the Process. It enables you to deal with the daily difficulties and disappointment that life throws up and emerge victorious.

## EmWave2

**www.heartmathstore.com/category/emWave2/**

If you have $169 to spare, this could be for you. It's a little piece of hardware, connected to software on your computer, that clips on your ear and transmits your pulse data, showing it as graphics and lights on the screen. It's a modern-day version of bio feedback. You can see at a glance if your heart rate is climbing and/or your breathing is getting out of balance.

The company also produce 'Inner Balance Trainer', a self-monitoring and training system for IOS devices. A bit less expensive at $99.

# CHAPTER 20
# USEFUL GADGETS

<br>

THE ONLY GADGET you really need is a good dry skin brush. That said, there are a few things that make life easier that you could buy, if you think you would make use of them.

## LEMON JUICER

I used to cut a new lemon in half each morning and squeeze it by hand into each glass of water through the day. When I bought a lemon juicer, I realized I had been a bit wasteful doing it by hand, as I extracted far more juice using the juicer.

I like the Amco Enameled Aluminum Lemon Squeezer[14] because it is beautiful and simple. I'm not usually a fan of aluminum products in the kitchen but this is one I've let slip through because it is so handy.

---

14 http://amzn.com/B0002V23BG

I also have the Magimix Juicer, which has a citrus juice attachment. I confess that I hardly ever use the attachment, because it is fiddly. I use the juicer for juicing vegetables daily, it sits on my kitchen counter but going the extra mile of taking off the top of the juicer and exchanging it for the citrus attachment is just too much! It may not be for you though.

If you prefer low-tech and simple, plastic lemon squeezers are very inexpensive and there is a lovely glass one[15] by Kitchen Craft for under $4.

# VITAMIX BLENDER[16]

I saw these for years on shopping channels and at shows before taking the leap and buying one. It was a big leap, they cost over $400! Wow, but I totted up the sums and it made sense. At that point I was using a blender twice a day, every day - a morning smoothie and nut milk. I burnt out a blender about every 6 months. I was spending around $30 on each, so I upped it to buy a better quality blender of around $60, thinking it would last longer. It didn't.

An American friend told me that her Mom had had a Vitamix for 30 years and it was still working. So I saved up and took advantage of an offer in my local Costco, where they were $50-off the regular price.

I can honestly say that it is one of the best things I have ever bought. I hate being ripped off and am careful what I buy but if my Vitamix did break, I would certainly buy another.

---

15 http://amzn.com/B000LCN1DA
16 http://amzn.com/B008H4SLV6

I used to have to sieve the nut milk but the Vitamix makes it so smooth that it doesn't need sieving. It's therefore more economical because it doesn't waste the bits of the almonds that used to end up in the sieve.

It makes smoothies with crushed ice that are deliciously thick and nourishing. I add all sorts of seeds to our smoothies and no-one would know as they are completely pulverized!

# REBOUNDER

People who see me walk - or try to walk - are often astonished that I can use a rebounder. It's because I don't jump on it, I bounce. I have a folding one that I keep in my kitchen and I use it for 5 minutes every morning. If I don't, my day tends not to go to plan as I am a lot less energized and coordinated. If I can find time later in the day, I will use it for a couple of minutes again.

I use mine next to a kitchen cupboard, so I can hold on lightly to steady myself if I start to lose my balance. The basic technique is very simple but you can get really clever on these things and get a great, all-round workout. Even just a gentle bounce is very stimulating - it actually exercises every cell in your body as they are raised by your bounce and pulled down again by gravity. Remember the internal pressure that moves lymph in and out of the ISF? We're talking about that sort of pressure here. Pressure that exercises you all over internally, not just moves the odd muscle here and there.

Rebounding is tremendous all-over exercise that really gets the lymph moving and makes you feel great.

I don't use rebounding DVDs, but I know people who like both Jason Vale's and Gunnar Peterson's.

# AIR WALKER

Due to my ankle problems, I have difficulty walking so the usual advice that health professionals give, to do more walking, is out for me. Pete Egoscue, the posture guy I mentioned earlier, recommends exercise that keeps the body in correct alignment, so I looked for something suitable. Enter the Air Walker. It exercises both arms and legs but is totally non-impact. The legs glide back and forth, with the feet pointing forward - they can't start drifting to the side! It is a big piece of equipment but folds up small enough to put in a cupboard or under a bed.

The Gazelle Edge[17] is a good one - I found mine for $20 on Ebay!

---

17 http://amzn.com/B0000AS7W2

# Appendix 1
## Contraindications For Skin Brushing

෴

D RY SKIN BRUSHING is a bit like an extremely effective massage. Therefore, the things that make massage a bad idea also make skin brushing a bad idea. These aren't mere suggestions - these are the things that insurance companies tell masseurs to avoid because they know that massage can make these problems worse and people could sue. So it is wise to listen to them!

These are:

**Cancer**

Brushing, like massage, improves lymphatic circulation and, as cancer can be spread via the lymphatic system, this means that brushing/massage are not a good idea. It may be that your doctor or oncologist says massage is OK - cancers vary - but if not, it is vital to follow their instructions.

## Diabetes

Get a medical expert's advice first.

## High blood pressure/Heart conditions

Brushing works on the blood vessels, which are already dealing with excess pressure. After checking with a medical expert, you may be allowed some very gentle massage, though. In that case, start with your hands and move onto very gentle, light brushing.

## Fractures/breaks

Stay away from the affected area but brushing other parts of the body can actually help the healing of the break by improving circulation. Muscle and tendon ruptures are also best avoided - pain will probably tell you that!

## Infection and/or Fever

Your body is working hard, often by turning up the temperature to kill some invaders (bacteria/virus). Don't make it work harder. Let the infection/fever burn out first.

## Inflammation or swelling

You don't want to brush over areas of inflammation or swelling as you could make them worse. This includes varicose veins, as discussed earlier, as well as hernias, growths, boils and other protrusions. You can brush around them but don't get too close. Certain types of arthritis cause almost permanent swelling in joints. Again, these are best avoided but you can brush the areas surrounding them.

## Open wounds/cuts

Stay away from the area until it is healed.

## Osteoporosis

If your bones are brittle your skin and connective tissues are often fragile too.

To sum up, **any** acute or chronic pain or illness should be a warning sign that you shouldn't do skin brushing or massage. Get medical advice first.

I know that all books that mention health or fitness topics say that you 'should consult your doctor before embarking on any...' blah, blah, and that most doctors aren't in the slightest bit interested in stuff like this, seeing it as unscientific and therefore ineffective. However, if you have any health condition you really should MAKE your doctor listen to you - perhaps write it down or show him/her this book - and double check that it is OK to stimulate your lymphatic system through skin brushing. Explain that it will also be stimulating your blood, lymph, immune systems, etc., which is very important if you have an auto-immune disorder (I do, and I've been given the go ahead to have massage/do skin brushing, but do check first as these conditions vary tremendously).

If you doctor does give you the go-ahead, just be careful to avoid brushing any affected or sensitive areas. You can still get the benefit of skin brushing even if you have to avoid one or two parts of your body.

Generally, if you have been told to avoid massage you should also avoid skin brushing. .

# Appendix 2
# FAQ About Skin Brushing

## ❦

## *Do I have to use a brush?*

No, but a brush will give you the best possible results. You can get some (but not all) of the benefits of skin brushing by using your hands (which will help lymph flow), a loofah (which will help exfoliation), or other device.

Don't be fooled by cosmetic companies which seem to offer a different device every year for helping cellulite, weight, or whatever. A brush is all you need and it will stimulate the lymphatic system without pressing down too hard on the initial lymph vessels.

## *Can I brush when I have a cold?*

Minor sniffles, yes, it's actually beneficial because it helps the immune system. If you get a fever, though, or feel 'chesty' you could have an infection and that's your body telling you quite loudly that you need rest and rehydration. Save the brushing for when you start to feel bored and irritated at all the lying around – that's your body telling you it's time to get moving.

## Do I have to brush in the morning?

No. People's schedules and family pressures vary and I understand that mornings can be particularly fraught. You can brush any time of day that suits you. The only difference is brushing in the evenings. If it's within an hour or two of bedtime, you will need to brush much more gently. Read the 'Super Relaxing Before Bed Brushing Routine' chapter.

## Will it make any difference if I don't shower after skin brushing?

No, if you don't have time it's fine. The idea of showering after skin brushing is to wash off the dead skin cells that the skin brushing dislodges. You can just wash them off later in the day when you do shower or bathe.

## Can I wash my brush?

Yes. It will reduce its lifespan slightly, as it will soften the bristles. Having said that, I've had my brush for over 20 years and it's still going strong, despite washing it regularly.

## My brush is way too stiff, it hurts no matter how gently I brush. What can I do?

Some brushes are stiffer than others. Generally, plant fiber brushes are better than artificial fibers. Try softening your brush's fibers by washing it in warm water a couple of times. Use it just on the palms of your hands and soles of your feet. They are tough enough to take it and it will help break in the brush. You can just use your hands to do the brushing movements on the rest of your body. That will get your body used to the movements and might help prepare the skin for the tougher brush later on! If you still find it too hard it might be time to try a different brush, sadly.

## How vigorously should I brush?

At first, not vigorously at all because you want to get used to the amount of pressure you can exert, and get your body used to the movements. After you're used to skin brushing you can start to experiment with the pressure and speed. Generally, you'll want to brush a little more vigorously if you're brushing in the mornings and much slower and more relaxed if you're brushing in the evenings – so you don't over-stimulate your system before bed.

## Can I brush if I have had lymph glands removed?

Possibly but you really need to get professional medical advice first. Even more importantly, you need to be sure that you are clear of cancer, or there is a danger of helping it travel around the body to other areas.

Manual lymphatic therapists often help patients who have had glands removed. They 'teach' the lymph to divert towards the nearest healthy lymph cluster.

## I LOVE skin brushing, I'm getting great benefits. Is it possible to do it too much though?

Yes. Twice a day is fine for a few weeks, more than that and you could start to irritate your skin. I would suggest cutting down to once a day if you want to brush daily forever, or a couple of times a week if you prefer to brush both morning and evening.

## *Can I brush if I have acne?*

Yes – it's a good idea. Just don't brush over any affected areas.

You do want to encourage lymphatic drainage, though, so brush all the parts of your body that don't have any spots. Rehydrating will also help, as will keeping a food diary to see if you can discover any food or lifestyle reactions. Dumping chemical cleansers and moisturizers can also be a breakthrough. Use simple grapeseed or almond oil to cleanse and moisturize. It makes your skin feel great and it will help reduce the inflammation.

# APPENDIX 3
# FOOD INTOLERANCE

ളെ

MANY YEARS AGO an old friend of mine had a baby who was badly intolerant to cow's milk. Well-meaning medics told her to gradually introduce milk a little a time into his diet to 'get him used to it'.

That made me want to scream – but I didn't have any qualifications at the time so didn't feel I should say anything. It just didn't seem right, though. It would be like introducing arsenic into your diet to try to develop a tolerance to it – not a good idea! She didn't want him to be different, to stand out in a negative way, so she went ahead with the gradual reintroduction of the foods he reacted to.

He's now an adult who can handle himself in any social situation. His health, however, isn't great. He looks swollen, puffy-faced and I gather he has digestive issues.

If you have ever been on a special diet, or had to avoid certain foods, you'll know how difficult it can be socially. There's cultural pressure to conform, to all eat the same. People who are a bit different bear the brunt of the annoyance of others.

Sometimes this comes from guilt – perhaps they are aware that their diet is less than optimal – but often it is just the natural instinct to eat like everyone else.

This can cause people to try to belong, food-wise, and ignore problems that they know are there.

It doesn't help that the media keep reporting on weird and wonderful diets that are popular with celebrities. These trendy diets are portrayed as 'faddy' because they suggest cutting out certain things.

'Wheat Belly' is one of the most popular of recent years. Written by a cardiologist, Dr William Davis, it is based on a diet that he discovered when experimenting with his patients' diets, trying to lower their blood sugar. He found that foods made from wheat flour raised blood sugar even more than sugar did. He advised his patients to remove wheat flour products (white and brown) from their diets and, not only did they get their blood sugar under control, they also lost weight. He went on to write his book based on these experiences.

Yet this man was pilloried in the press because his book was seen as another fad diet. Who would you rather believe? The ever changing press or a learned, qualified, dedicated doctor?

Dr Davis is convinced that wheat flour products are the cause of much disease and distress. He has earned our attention.

I was mildly aware of 'Wheat Belly' when my good friend and highly qualified nutritionist, Janet Matthews (who trained with Patrick Holford of the Institute of Optimum Nutrition) released a book containing excellent gluten-free recipes.

I implemented her advice to give up gluten products and make up lots of recipes from her book. I not only lost over a stone in a few weeks, I stopped suffering from digestive problems and found that my concentration and productivity improved. I'm convinced that gluten had been having a serious [negative] effect on me.

During Christmas some gluten-filled foods crept back into my diet. The result was digestive disaster (I won't go any further into that, if you're a sufferer you'll understand and if you're not you really don't want to know!) but also, surprisingly, reduced mental functioning. I experienced frequent dizzy spells, completely lacked concentration, and just couldn't stop crying.

I put it down to empty nest syndrome – my son having just got married – but the nest wasn't completely empty, my daughter is still at home, and it seemed more than that. After going gluten-free again, the symptoms lifted.

Now we know that gluten causes digestive problems in those who are susceptible/intolerant to it but not many people realize the gut/brain connection. There is, in effect, a second brain in the gut – in fact more serotonin (the 'happy' hormone that the popular antidepressant Prozac affects) is made in the gut than in the brain. 90% of the body's supply of serotonin is found in the gut, in special cells that line the gut (called enterochromaffin or Kulchitsky cells).

Gluten, in Latin, means 'glue' and that's just the effect it has on many people. It glues up the lining of the intestine so you can no longer absorb enough nutrients, leading to numerous problems.

If your enterochromaffin cells are bunged up with sticky gluten, they're not able to produce and process serotonin properly. Could this be why IBS is often accompanied by depression? Why people with food intolerance often suffer from fatigue and apathy?

## Becoming A Detective – With Team Members

What if you're intolerant to lots of things? What if you've cut out the usual culprits – corn, wheat, dairy – and you still have horrible health problems?

Then you need to become a detective, and detectives work best with other professionals. You're the expert on your own body, your own symptoms, but you need the advice of other experts too on things like nutrition, diagnosis, herbal medicines, etc.

The danger of becoming your own diagnostician and cutting out lots of things from your diet is that you'll go further down the road to malnutrition. If you're already intolerant, you won't be absorbing all the nutrients from the food you are eating, cutting out more could make it much worse.

Here are a few steps you could take to find out your particular food problems:

1. Start keeping a [brutally honest] food diary. This is absolutely essential. You need to make a note of what you eat, quantity, and any effects you noticed afterwards. The easiest way is to make a note of how you're feeling every time you eat something. If you're not a fan of writing you could substitute taking photos of your food. The app **Eatly** is a way of recording a photo food diary on a smartphone (IOS or Android).

2. Book an appointment with a qualified nutritionist, ideally one who has experienced food intolerance themselves. Show him/her your food diary sheets. These will help in diagnosis, but there will probably be other forms to fill in to help get a full picture of how food is affecting you.

3. Be prepared to cut out certain foods on the nutritionist's advice. It isn't easy. It's common to fall early on and 'give

in' to old comfort foods. This is going to be something of an endurance test.

4. Determine to act healthily in order to get healthy. When you're in peak condition it's easy to choose healthy foods because your body isn't craving all sorts of rubbish. Act now *as if* you are a really healthy person who doesn't like junk food. It can really help.

5. Take supplements as recommended by your nutritionist or holistic doctor. They can get you over cravings and difficulties withdrawing from foods you have become dependent upon – which often is the very ones you are intolerant to. If you are giving up some food groups you may need to stay on supplements, certain for the first few months while your body adapts to the new regime.

Experts vary in opinion on whether food intolerance tests are worth taking. Nutritionists who work for the food intolerance labs – unsurprisingly – support them! Skeptics point out that one person's blood sample sent to three different labs will come back with three different lists of foods to avoid. If you can't afford a test, then comfort yourself with that fact!

Some people need tests in order to be able to stick to what can turn out to be quite a restrictive diet, though. If that's you and you can afford it, then go ahead and get yourself tested – it certain won't do any harm.

If you find you are intolerant to wheat, you might want to read *Really Healthy Gluten Free Living* by Janet Matthews. She is horrified at the ingredients in gluten free foods in supermarkets and health food stores - generally, the first ingredient is sugar. It's better, if you can, to make your own. Her book is full of recipes to do just that.

## Low Budget Detective Work

If you are on a restricted income and in despair at ever reclaiming your health, there is a low budget method to determine if you are reacting to certain foods.

This isn't scientifically approved and I'm sure most experts would raise an eyebrow or two at it. However, if you don't have any other options you're probably – like I was – willing to try most things as long as they aren't going to harm you. This certainly won't.

Don't do this if you think you have an allergy to the food – which can be life-threatening – only do it if you suspect an intolerance. Certainly don't try it with food/drink that you have been told to avoid by a professional.

Here it is:

1.  Avoid the suspect food for at least two days, preferably two weeks.
2.  Get a large portion of it and sit down to relax for 15 minutes (have someone serve it to you after the 15 minutes if it's a food that you prefer hot!).
3.  Take your pulse and write it down (be sure to write each reading that follows down as well).
4.  Eat the food and take your temperature immediately after eating.
5.  Take your pulse again 30 minutes later and 30 minutes after that. So you're taking 3 readings after eating the suspect food, each 30 minutes apart.

Read through your readings for the whole day, or several days if you can and have a few different foods to test.

You may notice pulse rate spikes after eating a food that your body reacts to. That's the food to give up.

Keeping these records so you can refer back to them will be very helpful later on when you start missing that food.

Food intolerance, far from being a fad, is a very real and damaging problem. It literally physically damages your gut lining, with all kinds of knock-on effects.

Don't think like the doctors of old and keep reintroducing the suspect food into your diet. Just accept that you're going to have to avoid it for perhaps six months while your gut lining heals. Then try reintroducing it in one large portion and doing the pulse test again. If you still react, give it another 3-6 months before repeating.

## Other Things To Test

You can use the pulse test for other things as well. I found I was reacting to a particular shampoo and a supplement I had been taking for some time.

In particular, test foods, drinks, and habits that you feel you can't do without. They're the first suspects on your list!

Consider testing your pulse before and after:

- ➤ Coffee, tea, cigarettes or whatever you use in the morning to pick you up – including healthy options such as green juices and smoothies.
- ➤ Supplements – you can become intolerant to one particular ingredient and therefore can switch to another.
- ➤ Using a cellphone.
- ➤ Using a computer or tablet.
- ➤ Watching television.

> ➤ Going on vacation. Sometimes we become intolerant to our home environments, perhaps because of something like damp or mold. If you find you always feel better on vacation, it may not just be due to the lack of stress, it could be environmental too.

It is very frustrating and can take some time to get to the bottom of multiple food intolerances. The good news is that finding and avoiding them for some months can give your body time to heal and you may be able to enjoy them again in future.

# ACKNOWLEDGMENTS

 ‎‪☙

THIS BOOK TOOK a long time to test, research, and write. I am grateful to the many people who have been a part of creating this new method of skin brushing, especially the ~~clients~~ friends whose feedback taught me more than I taught them.

Grateful thanks, as always, to my family for their continual support and for putting up with my regular absences and my distracted presence when I am around.

Thanks go especially to my teachers in the fields of aromatherapy, anatomy, physiology, and nutrition: Marian Delgaudio Mak, Patrick Holford, Dr Eric Berg, Valerie Ann Worwood, Maggie Tisserand, and Kitty Campion – and other wellness professionals whose work I follow: Dr Joel Kahn, Phil Parker, Janey Lee Grace, Kris Carr, Dr Joel Kahn, Dr Ross Trattler, Vani Hari (the Food Babe), Dr Joseph Mercola, Jason Vale, and Joe Cross.

Huge thanks to the health professionals who helped put me back together when I was in pieces and kept me going since, including but not limited to: Mr David Vaughan (surgeon), Miss Colette Balmer (surgeon), Kay Atkinson (osteopath), Jane Vigon (Lightning Process therapist), Jonathan Hall (physiotherapist).

Thanks and kudos too to Nancy Hendrickson and the team at Green Pony Press, Inc., who published the first imprint of this book. Writers always think they have a reasonable grasp of the English language until they get the proof copies back! I'm very grateful for and in awe of my support team.

Special thanks to Cathy Presland for starting me on the road to publishing rather than talking about publishing! Her friendship and guidance helped this book become a reality.

During the course of writing this book a number of things happened: the deaths of Rosemary Jeffrey, Eileen Campbell, and my beloved dog, Ailsa; the demise of my precious Macbook; my mother's diagnosis of and treatment for cancer; some drastic home problems, including the dining room ceiling falling in and the bathroom springing a leak that took nine months to locate.

These events all happened within weeks of each other and I experienced a crisis, finding myself depressed and unable to concentrate and be creative. So I took on the help of an old friend, who has now become a celebrated business coach. Huge, eternally grateful thanks to Keith Wells of Keith Wells Associates for helping me get my brain back into gear, my time management sorted out, my creative juices flowing again, and for helping me enlarge my boundaries.

I am very glad that I eventually - six months late - managed to finish this book, because I think it needed writing. I have been on a lifelong quest for health and I wish I had discovered my new method of skin brushing a long time ago. It is my hope and prayer that this book helps you on your personal quest for mental, physical, and spiritual health.

*Mia x*

# INDEX

CʒຂꙨ

# ABOUT THE AUTHOR

ೞ

MIA CAMPBELL, I.I.H.H.T., is an experienced aromatherapist and health coach. She was born in Lancashire in the UK and treats private clients in the North-West of England.

Mia is engaged to Andrew and has two adult children. She enjoys playing and writing music, field archery, and swimming. She is about to embark on an extended road trip in a 5th Wheeler around the US and Canada and will be blogging about it at:

**www.britsinabus.info**

One of Mia's other interest is psychology and its effect on health. She has written a guide to understanding your own health personality and you can download it free at:

**http://yourhealthpersonality.subscribemenow.com**

Made in the USA
Middletown, DE
01 June 2015